Educational, Medical and Advisory Provision for Children with Epilepsy in Ireland

By
Joyce Senior B.Ed. (Hons.) Ph.D.

Forewords
by
Dr. B.J. Spelman
Education Department, University College Dublin

Professor Harry McMahon
University of Ulster

Mike Glynn
Chief Executive, Brainwave, The Irish Epilepsy Association

Parents' Comment on the Present Study

"On a personal note we are delighted this survey is being carried out. Epilepsy is still greatly misunderstood by our generation. Hopefully our children will have a better understanding and not be so afraid of the condition. Explaining our feelings etc. was particularly painful but this survey can only help our little girl and give her the best possible future which is all we would wish for her. Thank you and good luck."

Dedicated to the Memory of my Brother,

Kenneth Senior
1956-1997

ACKNOWLEDGEMENTS

This study was conducted as a doctoral research thesis at the Education Department, University College Dublin (National University of Ireland, Dublin) over the period September 1998 - April 2001. It was carried out under the expert supervision of Dr. Brendan Spelman, clinical and educational child psychologist, my academic supervisor at the Education Department, UCD, to whom I would like to express my profound gratitude for his invaluable advice, direction, inspiration and support.

I would also like to take this opportunity to gratefully acknowledge the contribution of the following people, without whom it would not have been possible to complete this study:

The staff of Brainwave, the Irish Epilepsy Association, and in particular Mr. Mike Glynn, Chief Executive, Ms. Geraldine Dunne, Information Officer/Counsellor, and Mr. Paul Sharkey, National Training and Communications Manager, who gave so freely of their time throughout the study, and without whose co-operation this research would not have been possible.

The Church of Ireland College of Education for the award of a Millennium Scholarship in support of the study.

The Irish National Teachers' Organisation for their interest in the thesis and their financial support. A particular word of thanks is due to Senator Joe O'Toole who, in his capacity as General Secretary of the I.N.T.O, co-launched the research findings in October 2001.

Dr. Deirdre McMackin, formerly senior clinical neuropsychologist in Beaumont Hospital, Dublin, and Dr. Bryan Lynch, consultant paediatric neurologist in The Children's Hospital, Temple Street, Dublin, for their constructive advice on the questionnaire.

Dr. Frank Besag for his expert opinions and advice, and for so kindly inviting me to St. Pier's Lingfield Medical Hospital, Surrey.

My family, for their continuous support of a study which was a constant, and often painful, reminder of our loss. A special word of thanks to my dear sister, Gwen Stanley, who has helped me in so many ways during the difficult times.

The parents of the children in the study who gave so willingly of their time, and without whose contribution this study would not have been possible.

FOREWORD

I am delighted and very privileged as academic supervisor to be asked to write the foreword to what is a seminal study in the field of epilepsy. This is the first study of the perinatal, developmental, educational and socio-cultural concomitance of epilepsy among schoolgoing children in the Republic of Ireland. It has important implications, not only for an enhanced understanding of the nature of epilepsy in familial and educational contexts, but also for the development of public policies in the areas of health, education and support services in general, as these relate to the condition of epilepsy.

A particularly satisfactory consequence of the study is the extent to which its recommendations are being adopted by the relevant Government Departments and voluntary associations in the Republic of Ireland, most notably by Brainwave, the Irish Epilepsy Association.

I wish the findings of the study the widest possible dissemination, not only among the relevant professionals, but also among teachers, for too many of whom children with epilepsy still constitute the Hidden Children in our education system.

Dr. B.J. Spelman BA, MA (Ed.), MSc. (Psych.)
Senior Lecturer,
Education Department, University College Dublin,
National University of Ireland, Dublin

FOREWORD

Parents of children with epilepsy everywhere in Ireland will welcome this important work by Dr. Joyce Senior. For those mothers and fathers who are living with the problems of being a parent of a child with epilepsy there will be reassurance that many others have had to go through similar difficulties. Some who have been down this hard road in the past will be pleased to see that at last what they went through has been acknowledged. Future parents whose children are born with or develop epilepsy will find this book a great source of information about their child's condition, a roadmap to the obstacles which they may encounter in bringing up their child and crucially, information on how to overcome these difficulties.

For all of us involved with Brainwave, the Irish Epilepsy Association, Joyce's book reminds us of what it is we are working towards, and points us firmly in the direction of trying to improve conditions for children with epilepsy and their families. In fact, for anyone anywhere with an interest in epilepsy, Joyce Senior's "Educational, Medical and Advisory Provision for Children with Epilepsy" is an indispensable source book and point of reference.

Mr. Mike Glynn,
Chief Executive,
Brainwave, the Irish Epilepsy Association

FOREWORD

This is an excellent study that breaks new ground in education research in Ireland. The stance taken is critical and analytical, the writing is fluent and excellent use is made of relevant literature from the United Kingdom, Europe and the United States of America as well as the Republic of Ireland. The first six chapters constitute an in-depth and comprehensive survey of factors contributing to an understanding of the educational, medical and advisory provision for children with epilepsy in the Republic of Ireland. Successive chapters consider the nature of epilepsy, historical and contemporary conceptions and beliefs about the condition, family responses and adjustments to its occurrence, factors affecting the educational and social adjustment of sufferers and the educational provision and legislative framework experienced by children with epilepsy in England and Ireland.

The methods used to identify a sample of parents of children with epilepsy and those employed to produce and administer the data collection instrument were entirely appropriate to the research aims and to the field conditions faced by the author. The limitations of the study are fully explored and acknowledged. Despite the fact that the sample of parents is relatively small, the data set created can nevertheless be considered to be the most comprehensive and potentially informative as yet produced in Ireland on epilepsy and its effects on children and their families.

The analysis of the data set is thorough and systematic and the results effectively presented in tabular and graphical form. Emerging from a critical discussion of the results, a fully justified set of recommendations is presented, couched in clear and direct terms that add weight to their import. The research report and its recommendations are then exposed to a mature professional working in the field, one well placed to judge their contemporary relevance and practicability. The account in the closing chapter that flows from this 'field testing' of the research of itself adds further credibility and authenticity to the work.

In all, the study is a work of considerable significance. It exhibits original and critical thinking and makes a substantial contribution to knowledge and scholarship.

Professor Harry McMahon,
University of Ulster

CONTENTS

LIST OF FIGURES

LIST OF TABLES

CHAPTER ONE

THE NATURE OF EPILEPSY

1.1 INTRODUCTION

This chapter begins with an overview of the meanings of the word epilepsy, both historically and in current usage. The definitions of the condition epilepsy which are used by various organisations and medical professionals are also examined. The terminology and classifications used to distinguish epilepsy and the varying types of seizures are then outlined. Following the classifications of epilepsy, the different types of seizures are identified. The aetiology of epilepsy and the factors which can trigger seizures are then considered. The chapter concludes with a consideration of the epidemiology of epilepsy.

1.2 THE WORD 'EPILEPSY'

McGovern (1985) comments that epilepsy, as a word, has probably caused more anxiety and heartache than almost any other word in medical parlance. It is a word that many people shy away from; it has overtones and undertones and it illustrates very clearly the truth of the old adage 'a little learning is a dangerous thing' because people often think they know what it means, when in fact they don't. She adds that it is really a practically useless word, because it is an umbrella term with many widely differing interpretations.

Epilepsy is a Greek word, derived from the verb epilambanein; epi means upon and lepsy is from the root lambano, meaning to seize (Mc Govern, 1985). The word epilepsy comes from the Greek word epilepsia, which means to be taken, grabbed, attacked, possessed or seized (Dam and Gram, 1986, O'Donohue, 1994). The image survived in the English word 'seizure'. An epileptic seizure may also be called an ictus, which originally meant a blow or a strike. The derived adjectives, post-ictal and interictal are often used to refer to behaviours during, after or between seizures (Lebrun, 1992).

The modern view of epilepsy originated in the work of the mid-nineteenth century neuroscientists, the most important among them being John Hughlings Jackson, who defined epilepsy as 'occasional, sudden, excessive, rapid and local discharges of grey matter' (Trimble and Reynolds, 1981). Building on this foundation, modern epileptologists have defined and redefined the various forms of clinical epilepsy. Engel (1995) states that at present, the word 'epilepsy' is used to refer to a class of epileptic disorders, defined as chronic neurological conditions characterised by recurrent epileptic seizures. Epileptic seizures, in turn, can be defined as the clinical manifestation of excessive and/or hypersynchronous, usually self-limited, abnormal activity of neurons, predominantly located in the cerebral cortex.

1.3 DEFINITIONS OF EPILEPSY

In their attempts to define epilepsy, many authors acknowledge that Hughlings Jackson's (1931) concept of a seizure as being due to 'an occasional, an excessive and a disorderly discharge of nerve tissue' is difficult to better (O'Donohue 1994, Sutherland and Eadie, 1980).

As the term 'The Epilepsies' suggests, there is no single disease 'epilepsy'. Rather, there is a group of disorders, the epilepsies, which appear to involve similar pathophysiological mechanisms which develop in different anatomical regions of the brain, have different aetiologies and are associated with different electroencephalographic appearances (Sutherland and Eadie, 1980).

According to the World Health Organisation, an epileptic seizure is the result of transient dysfunction of part, or all of the brain due to excessive discharge of an hyperexcitable population of neurons, causing sudden and transitory phenomena of motor, sensory, autonomic or psychic nature (Gastaut, 1973).

Mc Govern (1985) states that medically, a person with epilepsy is someone who is subject to recurrent interruptions of brain function, due to sudden, disorderly nerve cell discharge. However, she adds that epilepsy is not a 'nervous' condition in the generally accepted sense of the word.

Sutherland and Eadie (1980) state that epilepsy is best regarded as a symptom, due to a commonly occurring type of brain dysfunction. It can be defined and regarded as a symptom due to excessive temporary neuronal discharging which results from intracranial or extracranial causes. Epilepsy is characterised by discrete episodes which tend to be recurrent, in which there is a disturbance of movement, sensation, behaviour, perception and/or consciousness.

In their review of epilepsy, Aird, Masland and Woodbury (1984) refer to epilepsy as a paroxysmal disturbance of central nervous system (CNS) function, which is recurrent, stereotyped in character, and associated with excessive neuronal discharge that is synchronous and self-limited.

Gastaut (1973) states that epilepsy is defined as a chronic brain disorder of various aetiologies characterised by recurrent seizures. Brainwave, the Irish Epilepsy Association, defines epilepsy as a condition characterised by a tendency to have recurring, spontaneous seizures. In their Teacher's Guide to Epilepsy (1992), it is stated that a seizure is "a brief and temporary disturbance of the brain function and the tendency of individuals to convulse can vary considerably. It is not a disease, nor is it contagious."

Sillanpaa et al. (1990) consider that usually two or more unprovoked seizures, with the minimum interval of more than 24 hours are defined as epilepsy. The definition implies exclusion of cases with a single seizure, febrile convulsions and other occasional seizures, progressive brain disorders, and metabolic diseases.

According to Hall and Smithson (1997), epilepsy is the most common serious neurological condition and is characterised by recurrent unprovoked seizures. Shorvran (1987) and Hopkins (1987) define epilepsy as a continuing tendency to seizures that are caused by paroxysmal discharge of cerebral neurons, resulting in a clinical event apparent to the subject, or an observer, or both.

In their education booklet, Epilepsy and Education (1995), the British Epilepsy Association states that epilepsy is "an established tendency for the brain to experience recurrent seizures in which total or partial consciousness may be lost. An epileptic seizure is caused by a brief disruption of brain function involving abnormal electrical activity in the nerve cells."

Mc Menamin and O'Connor Bird (1997), in their Parent's Guide to Epilepsy, define epilepsy as a "recurrent, episodic, uncontrolled electrical discharge from the brain. It is the term for recurrent, unprovoked seizures or convulsions."

1.4   CLASSIFICATIONS

The terminology and classification of epilepsy have evolved over many years, creating a profusion of interchangeable and confusing descriptive terms. In recent decades, there has been an increasing realisation of the need for a common, international terminology and classification of seizure disorders. This is of the utmost importance for the communication and exchange of ideas between people interested in such disorders, and a prerequisite for comparison of results in therapy and research.

In 1964, an international committee was convened by the International League Against Epilepsy (ILAE) to formulate a comprehensive classification of epileptic seizures which would include the type of clinical seizure, the type of EEG seizure, the interictal EEG expression and the anatomical substrate, as well as the aetiology of the seizure and the age of the patient. Arising from this, a classification known as the International Classification of Epileptic Seizures was published (Gastaut, 1970).

Seizures were classified as:
1. Partial, or those beginning locally
2. Generalised, or those which are bilaterally symmetrical and without local upset. These may be convulsive or non-convulsive in nature.
3. Unilateral seizures
4. Unclassifiable seizures

This classification was revised in 1981 (Commission on Classification and Terminology of the ILAE, 1981). The main criticism of this revised classification has been that it has abandoned the use of some time-honoured terms, e.g. generalised tonic-clonic seizure instead of grand mal, absence instead of petit mal, complex partial seizure instead of temporal lobe or psychomotor seizure, myoclonic or atonic instead of minor motor seizure. However, O'Donohue (1994) believes that these terms have been used in an ambiguous manner in the past, the worst example being the use of the term 'petit mal' to describe any seizure other than 'grand mal', and also the application of the term to all varieties of absence attacks.

In 1985 this classification was supplemented by a classification of epilepsies and epileptic syndromes. In 1989, the Commission on Classification proposed a new International Classification of Epilepsies, Epileptic Syndromes and Related Seizure Disorders (Commission on Classification and Terminology of the ILAE, 1985, 1989). The International Classification of Epileptic Seizures (ICES) uses two major divisions. The first one is based on the presumed anatomic localization of seizure onset, that is, generalized versus localization-related (focal, local, partial) epilepsies. The second division considers epilepsies to be the consequence of a known or suspected structural or metabolic disorder (symptomatic); a hidden or occult disorder (cryptogenic); and those without presence of discerning aetiology (idiopathic).

International Classification of Epileptic Seizures (abbreviated by Egg-Olofsson, 1990)

I PARTIAL (FOCAL, LOCAL) SEIZURES

<u>A</u> Simple partial seizures (consciousness not impaired)
1. With motor symptoms
2. With somatosensory or special sensory symptoms (simple hallucinations, e.g. tingling, light flashes, buzzing)
3. With autonomic symptoms or signs (including epigastric sensation, pallor sweating, flushing, piloerection and pupillary dilation)
4. With psychic symptoms (disturbance of higher cerebral function) These symptoms rarely occur without impairment of consciousness and are much more commonly experienced as complex partial seizures.

<u>B</u> Complex partial seizures (with impairment of consciousness; may sometimes begin with simple symptomatology)
1. Simple partial onset followed by impairment of consciousness
2. With impairment of consciousness at onset

<u>C</u> Partial seizures evolving to secondarily generalised seizures (these may be generalised tonic-clonic, tonic, or clonic).
1. Simple partial seizures (A) evolving to generalised seizures
2. Complex partial seizures (B) evolving to generalised seizures
3. Simple partial seizures evolving to complex partial seizures, evolving to generalised seizures

II GENERALISED SEIZURES (Convulsive or Non-Convulsive)

A 1. Absence seizures
   2. Atypical absences
B Myclonic seizures; Myclonic jerks (single or multiple)
C Clonic seizures
D Tonic seizures
E Tonic-clonic seizures
F Atonic seizures (Astatic)
G Combinations of the above may occur (e.g. B and F, B and D)

III UNCLASSIFIED EPILEPTIC SEIZURES

IV ADDENDUM

International Classification of Epilepsies and Epileptic Syndromes and Related Disorders
(abbreviated by Egg-Olofsson, 1990)

1   Localisation-related (focal, local, partial) epilepsies and syndromes
1.1   Idiopathic (with age-related onset)
1.2   Symptomatic, e.g. simple partial, complex partial.
1.3   Cryptogenic

2   Generalised epilepsies and syndromes
2.1   Idiopathic (with age-related onset: listed in order of age) e.g. childhood absence, tonic-clonic
     wakening, juvenile myoclonic epilepsy
2.2   Cryptogenic or symptomatic (in order of age)
2.3   Symptomatic e.g. infantile spasms, Lennox-Gastaut syndrome

3   Epilepsies and syndromes, undetermined whether focal or generalised
3.1   With both generalised and focal seizures
3.3   Without unequivocal generalised or focal features All cases with generalised tonic-clonic
     seizures in which clinical and EEG findings do not permit classification as clearly generalised
     or localisation-related, such as in the cases of sleep-grand mal (GTCS), are considered not to
     have unequivocal generalised or focal features.

4   Special Syndromes
4.1   Situation related seizures

1.5   TYPES OF SEIZURES
1.5.1 Introduction
In an effort to arrive at an internationally accepted terminology for seizures, a French doctor, Henri Gastaut, redefined the names given to various types of seizures and grouped them under the headings 'generalised' and 'partial' (McGovern, 1985). There are many types of seizures and a person may have more than one type, but the pattern of seizures tends to remain relatively constant. The type of seizure depends on the part of the brain which is affected. If the whole brain is affected, the seizure is known as 'generalised' and there may be an impairment or loss of consciousness, however brief. When only part of the brain is involved, the seizure is known as 'partial' (focal), and consciousness, though affected, may not necessarily be lost. Although epilepsy is usually classified by seizure type, it can also be classified by syndromes. In an information booklet, Seizures (1992), Brainwave, the Irish Epilepsy Association, states that the ILAE has published a list of epileptic syndromes, the use of which should be encouraged. According to Hall and Smithson (1997), terms such as grand mal and petit mal should no longer be used because they inaccurately describe seizures and are open to misuse.

1.5.2 Generalised Seizures
In generalised seizures, both hemispheres of the brain are involved from the start of the seizure and consciousness is characteristically impaired. There are three common sorts of generalised seizures: tonic-clonic, myoclonic and absence seizures.

1. Tonic-Clonic Seizures (previously known as grand mal or major seizures), are the commonest generalised seizure type. This is what most people think of when they hear of epilepsy or the word 'seizure'. The seizure starts with the tonic phase in which the muscles contract and the body falls to the ground and becomes rigid. The chest muscles contract and the expulsion of air in the lungs often produces a strange cry as the person falls down unconscious. Their breathing may be irregular and their face may look pale, with a bluish tinge around the lips due to lack of oxygen. They may let out strange sounds, dribble, produce pink, blood-tinged saliva,

bite their tongue or be incontinent. This tonic phase lasts only for a few seconds and is followed by a phase in which the muscles relax and contract, producing jerking movements that are often rhythmical, according to the rhythmic discharge of the brain cells. This is known as the clonic phase, hence the name sometimes given to this type of seizure is a tonic-clonic seizure. This phase, which may go on for several minutes, is often accompanied by the frothing of excess saliva on the lips and a sound like a groan or grunt, which is entirely involuntary. If the tongue has been bitten in the fall the saliva may be blood-flecked. The convulsions gradually subside and the movements become less vigorous. When they cease, colour and breathing return to normal but the patient remains unconscious because the brain is temporarily exhausted. After the convulsion, a post-ictal (confusion) phase lasting 20-60 minutes follows, during which the patient may be confused and exhibit features of automatism and is likely to be sleepy, prior to regaining full consciousness.

2. Absence Seizures (previously called petit mal), fall into two categories; typical and atypical.
   a) Typical Seizure: This type of seizure has a sudden onset and finish, and altered consciousness, with or without automatisms or jerks. It affects only the part of the brain concerned with consciousness and is usually found only in children. There is a loss, or clouding of consciousness for a brief period of time, usually 10 to 20 seconds, often less. There is no movement, except perhaps a flickering of the eyelids and as soon as consciousness returns the child continues with what he or she was doing before the attack. Both the child and the carers may be unaware that anything has happened. The important aspect, in connection with this type of seizure, is that, although the child does not fall, he is in fact unconscious and therefore unable to receive messages, either visual or oral, because he is absent for the duration of the seizure. For this reason the condition is often mistaken for 'day-dreaming' or 'switching off'. Onlookers may not realise that the child who misses part of a sentence, or who doesn't respond when spoken to, may be having an absence seizure. This can lead to learning difficulties and even to psychosocial problems, as some children can have hundreds of absences in a day. Switching in and out of what is going on this frequently can be very confusing for a child, who may find it difficult to keep up at school. Instead of 'two plus two is four, and four plus two is six', the child may hear 'two plus two...six' and will not understand what is wrong when corrected. Parents and teachers may get impatient with the child, who will be completely at a loss as to what she has done to provoke this (Mc Menamin and O'Connor-Bird, 1997).
   (b) Atypical Seizure: This type of seizure has a less abrupt onset and cessation of consciousness.

3. Myoclonic Seizures
   The generalised myoclonic epilepsies which occur between the ages of one to six years form another age-related group of epilepsies with many similarities to infantile spasms. In myoclonic seizures there are myoclonic jerks or abrupt jerking of the limbs, accompanied by a loss of consciousness, which may be brief or followed by a tonic-clonic seizure. In their information booklet, Seizures (1992), Brainwave, the Irish Epilepsy Association, state that these often happen within a short time of waking up, either on their own or with other forms of generalised seizures. These are uncommon and often misdiagnosed. There is usually a strong family history. Frequently, there is an associated variable degree of mental handicap. The long-term outlook is uncertain and recovery from the more severe cases is rare (O'Connor et al. 1992).

1.5.3 Partial Seizures
These may be simple or complex, depending on whether consciousness is unaltered or impaired. Partial seizures are also known as focal or localisation-related and are the second most common form of seizures (Hopkins, 1983). In this type of seizure, the disturbances in brain activity begins in or involves a distinct or part area of the brain, so the person remains fully conscious. Many different parts of the brain can be affected and the nature of these seizures is usually determined by the function of the part of the brain involved. There are basically three types of partial seizures; simple partial, complex partial and secondarily generalised.

1   Simple Partial Seizures, sometimes known as 'focal', involve parts of the brain that have a simple function. If it starts in the part of the brain that controls movement, for example, it may show itself as a twitching in the thumb, or at the corner of the mouth. Consciousness is not impaired and the seizure is confined to either rhythmical twitching of one limb or part of a limb, or to unusual sensations such as pins and needles in a distinct part of the body. Often the seizure spreads to the hand, the arm and the entire side of the body; the left side if the right side of the brain is affected, and vice versa. If seizures spread to involve areas of the brain concerned with consciousness, simple partial seizures often progress to other types of partial seizures, or to a generalised seizure. When this happens the earlier symptoms can serve as a warning and are known as an aura. Motor (Jacksonian), Sensory and Rolandic (commonest childhood epilepsy) are examples of simple partial seizures. Rolandic is a simple partial seizure, often with secondary generalisation. It is probably the commonest epilepsy of childhood and seems to be caused by a temporary functional disturbance in the brain. The usual age of onset is between seven and ten years of age. The seizures typically occur during sleep, often becoming secondarily generalised, producing a tonic-clonic seizure. The prognosis is excellent, with or without drug treatment (O'Connor, 1992).

2. Complex Partial Seizures: These also start as a focal discharge in the part of the brain which is more complicated. The parts of the brain involved are under the temples and are called the temporal lobes. They are concerned with complicated movements like fastening buttons, hooks or eyes or putting on a jacket or dress. The temporal lobes also have a close connection with emotions, memory and consciousness. Complex partial seizures are the commonest type of partial seizure (previously called temporal lobe epilepsy). The seizure usually starts as a simple partial seizure, for example with an aura, and then the patient becomes inattentive. Impaired consciousness lasts longer than in a childhood absence (minutes rather than seconds) and can be accompanied by stereotypical behaviour, such as grimacing, sucking, chewing, plucking at their clothes, fumbling with buttons, smacking the lips, swallowing repeatedly, wandering around as if drunk, or undressing. Such actions, known as automatisms last less than five minutes. The post-ictal period of confusion can be prolonged and the person will have no clear recollection of their movements or actions (Hall and Smithson, 1997).

3. Secondarily Generalised Seizure If the discharge spreads, either of the above may progress to become a generalised convulsion called secondarily generalised seizure.

1.5.4 Status Epilepticus
Status epilepticus is the term applied to a single epileptic seizure of more than 30 minutes duration, or a series of seizures, during which function is not regained between ictal events, in a period lasting more than 30 minutes (Hall and Smithson, 1997). This type of seizure requires prompt treatment because when a convulsion is prolonged there is always a danger of complication, such as brain damage from lack of oxygen, or vomiting with aspiration of vomit into the lungs. People with various types of epilepsy may develop status epilepticus. If a patient with tonic-clonic seizures develops status epilepticus, it is known as convulsive status epileticus, the most common type.

Children with myoclonic epilepsy may also develop status epilepticus. This may take the form of continuous or intermittent absences, accompanied by brief twitching of muscles or myoclonic jerks and by head nods and akinetic or drop attacks. Occasionally, children with absence seizures (or petit mal) will develop status epilepticus. This is known as non-convulsive status epilepticus because there are no jerks or abnormal movements (McMenamin and O'Connor-Bird 1997).

1.5.5 Febrile Convulsions
Febrile convulsions are epileptic seizures precipitated by fever, arising from infection outside the nervous system, occurring in a child aged from six months to five years who is otherwise normal (Verity, 1995). The diagnosis is made from the history, as the seizure is usually over before the doctor sees the child. The risk of significant sequelae seems minimal from large population studies. However, children who are neurologically or developmentally abnormal or whose febrile convulsions are focal, recur within 24 hours, or last for more than 15 minutes, are more likely to subsequently develop epilepsy (Hall and Smithson, 1997).

1.5.6 Nocturnal Seizures

Nocturnal seizures tend to occur, either within the first few hours after going to sleep, mainly during sleep, or one to two hours before the usual awakening time, particularly during lighter sleep. Seizures occurring a few minutes to about one hour after awakening, so-called early morning seizures, can be included in this category. Many nocturnal seizures undoubtedly go unrecognised or unreported. Not surprisingly, when parents go to see a doctor after their child has a nocturnal fit, it will probably not be the very first one. Diagnostic features of nocturnal seizures include, for example, a witnessed focal or generalised tonic or clonic attack, waking with a bitten tongue, waking with a disordered bed, and post-ictal phenomena such as headache or Todd's paresis (Egg-Olofsson, 1985).

1.5.7 Flicker Seizures

According to Egg-Olofsson (1985) flicker or photic-induced seizures are attacks provoked by flickering or sudden flashing of light. They may occur in children with different types of epilepsy, or may be the only manifestation of a seizure disorder. Photosensitivity is age and gender dependent and also related to genetic factors. The median age for the occurrence of photic-induced seizures is 11-15 years, with a predominance of girls. The ratio of girls to boys is about 3:2. With respect to genetic factors, photosensitivity has been observed in more than one family member.

Television is the commonest precipitant of seizures, usually provoking a tonic-clonic seizure, sometimes preceded by myoclonic jerking. The use of repetitive flickering and of strobe lighting at discos are also possible trigger mechanisms for photic-induced seizures.

1.6 AETIOLOGY

There are many causes for epilepsy and it may begin at any age. Any person's brain has the capacity to produce a seizure if the circumstances are appropriate. Most brains are not likely to do this spontaneously and can therefore be said to have high 'seizure threshold' or high resistance to seizures. Individuals vary as to their threshold and in some individuals the existing seizure threshold may be lowered if the brain is subject to unusual stimulation, such as some drugs, certain frequencies of flickering lights, or injury. In an information booklet, Explaining Epilepsy (1992), Brainwave, the Irish Epilepsy Association state that if the injury is severe e.g. due to a road accident, infection, birth trauma, stroke or tumour, then epilepsy may develop as a consequence.

Some people just appear to have a highly sensitive brain i.e. a low seizure threshold. However, epilepsy can result from brain damage caused before or after birth. In many children no actual cause is identified. Although there is a malfunction in the brain, there is no actual brain damage or brain disease. This is the most common type of epilepsy, sometimes called idiopathic.

Many people are surprised to learn that most individuals are not born with epilepsy. Although some types of epilepsy are inherited or are caused by difficult births, where too little oxygen reaches the brain during delivery, more cases of epilepsy are caused by experiences during one's lifetime. Head injury, alcoholism, ingesting of poisons, including illegal drugs, extremely poor nutrition, strokes, brain tumors, prolonged high fever or brain illness and other injuries and diseases affecting the brain can all cause epilepsy.

According to Sander et al. (1990), no cause is found in the majority of cases of epilepsy (61%). Hauser (1978) states that generally 65-70% of the cases have unknown aetiology, while Chadwick (1990) says that some 70% of epileptic disorders are idiopathic. Hopkins (1995), however, maintains that in some cases there is an identifiable cause and the most notable ones are identified below.

Genetic/Hereditary Factors

O'Donohue (1994) notes that one of the questions asked most frequently about epilepsy is, "Is it inherited?" The fear of inheriting epilepsy has been present from earliest times and in all cultures. It is closely linked with the prejudice that many people have about individuals suffering from epilepsy. Much repressive legislation prohibiting marriages, prescribing sterilisation and limiting immigration has resulted. There is no doubt that in some types of epilepsy, heredity plays a significant role. Some forms of epilepsy, such as absence seizures, generalised tonic-clonic seizures of the idiopathic variety and photosensitive epilepsy have a strong hereditary basis (McMenamin and O'Connor Bird, 1997). Siblings of patients with absence seizures and typical EEG changes more often have the same EEG changes compared to controls. Monozygotic twins more often have the same spike and wave EEG pattern than dizygotic twins (Leviton and Cowan, 1982). Berkovic et al. (1998) studied 253 twin pairs in whom one or both reported seizures. They concluded that genetic factors are particularly important in the generalised epilepsies but also play a role in the partial epilepsies.

Genetic factors can act by causing the transmission of diseases, of which epileptic seizures may be a symptom. There are over 100 single gene disorders which may have epilepsy as a symptom, and most also have other gross clinical characteristics (McKusick, 1983). Together, however, they account for less than 2% of cases of epilepsy. Examples include autosomal dominant disorders such as tuberose sclerosis and neuro-fibromatosis, recessively inherited disorders such as the various degenerative lipid storage disorders of the nervous system and disorders of amino acid and carbohydrate metabolism, as well as some X-linked conditions such as Menkes' Syndrome. Seizures may also occur in clinical syndromes caused by chromosomal anomalies such as Down's Syndrome, and in syndromes due to sex chromosomal abnormalities (O'Donohue, 1994).

The prediction of risks for the offspring of individuals who have epilepsy also depends on the nature of the parental epilepsy. For example, the incidence of seizures in the offspring of parents with absence seizures is much higher than in the offspring of parents with other seizure types. Hauser and Anderson (1986) state that the overall incidence of epilepsy in the offspring, when one parent is affected, is about four per cent. When both parents are affected, it rises to ten per cent or more. If there are more than two family members affected, the risks are greater still. Unexplained is the fact that the children of mothers with epilepsy are more likely to develop epilepsy than are children of fathers with epilepsy. However, O'Donohue (1985) reports that the overall risk to a child of developing epilepsy when one parent has epilepsy is 2%-3%. Where both parents have epilepsy, it is approximately 25%. O'Connor et al. (1992), believe that the risk appears to be highest when epilepsy occurs at an early age in patients with idiopathic epilepsy, absence seizures or previous family history, particularly in the mother. With febrile convulsions and 'petit mal', genetic factors are of paramount importance, but they play a much less significant role in partial epilepsy and in some of the serious epileptic syndromes of infancy and early childhood e.g. infantile spasms.

Racial Factors
Racial factors seem to play a role, as whites more often than blacks have infantile spasms, primary generalised epilepsy, benign Rolandic epilepsy and Lennox-Gastaut syndrome, but not temporal and frontal lobe epilepsy (Santiago and Niedermeyer, 1988).

Congenital Abnormalities
Any congenital abnormality of the brain may lead to seizure activity and some of these abnormalities may be inherited. The Sturge Weber syndrome, tuberose sclerosis or neurfibromatosis are examples of this. Some abnormalities are now thought to be due to neuronal migration. Hippocampal sclerosis is an abnormality associated with temporal lobe epilepsy (Hopkins, 1995).

Prenatal and Perinatal Factors
Hopkins (1995) cautions that care must be taken when making the assumption of epilepsy occurring as a result of injury. Studies by Nelson and Ellenberg (1987) in the US and Ross et al. (1980) conclude that labour and delivery factors appear to contribute little to the subsequent development of childhood epilepsy. Maldevelopment of an intact nervous system, rather than damage at birth, appears to be a more common mechanism. Mc Govern (1985), however, comments that epilepsy may arise before birth as a result of a faulty distribution of substances in the foetus. It may also arise as a result of difficult birth causing some damage to brain cells.

In studies from Iceland (Gudmundsson, 1966) and Norway (Krohn, 1961), difficulties in delivery were regarded as constituting the most important aetiological factor. In a Finnish study

(Rantakallio and von Wendt, 1986), a cohort of 12,000 children were prospectively followed for 14 years. In the children with epilepsy no cause could be found in 57%, in 9% of cases it was due to prenatal causes, in 18% of cases it was due to perinatal causes and in 16% it was due to postnatal causes. When comparing risk factors in healthy children and children with epilepsy, prenatal factors (e.g. degenerative CNS disease, CNS malformation) formed the highest relative risks. Prematurity and low birth weight did not seem to be important risk factors. Similar findings are reported from an American study of 54,000 deliveries between 1959 and 1966 (Nelson and Ellenberg, 1987). They commented that, among the hundreds of prenatal and perinatal factors which were explored as predictors of childhood epilepsy, the principal predictors identified were congenital malformations of the foetus (cerebral and non-cerebral), a family history of neurological disorders (epilepsy or mental retardation in the mother, epilepsy or motor deficits in a sibling) and neonatal seizures.

For complex partial seizures a population-based case control study (Rocca et al. 1987a) showed that prenatal or perinatal factors were of no importance, with the exception of neonatal convulsions and babies that were small for gestational age at birth. Furthermore, seizure disorder in the mother, febrile seizures, cerebral palsy, head trauma and viral encephalitis were significantly more common in the patients. Risk factors for generalised tonic-clonic seizures investigated in the same way indicated convulsions in the mother, febrile seizure and head trauma. For absence seizures, the occurrence of febrile convulsions was the only factor significantly more common in patients compared to controls (Rocca et al.,1987c).

Severe Head Injury or Trauma
Late post-traumatic epilepsy is particularly likely after a depressed skull fracture, injury causing a dural tear, focal neurological signs or a long post-traumatic amnesic episode, especially if seizures occur in the first week after trauma (Hopkins, 1995).

Mc Menamin and O'Connor-Bird (1997) state that post traumatic epilepsy, or seizures following severe head injury, can occur at the time of the injury or even up to two years or more afterwards. A severe head trauma which causes direct injury to the brain is usually accompanied by loss of consciousness. Many people have other neurological problems following a severe head injury, including post-traumatic headaches, behaviour problems, learning difficulties and physical disabilities. They add that minor head injuries, even those involving hairline fractures, do not cause post-traumatic epilepsy.

Infections of the Brain
Any disease or disorder that affects the brain can result in epilepsy. The two main groups of infectious agents that may affect the brain are viruses and bacteria. Viruses may cause viral meningitis or encephalitis. A not uncommon brain infection, Herpes Encephalitis produced by the herpes virus, often results in epilepsy, but there are usually other signs of brain damage.

Common types of meningitis caused by bacteria include haemophilus meningitis, meningococcal meningitis and pneumococal meningitis (McMenamin and O'Connor-Bird, 1997). Hopkins (1995) states that patients with bacterial meningitis can develop seizures during the acute phase (30%), or up to five years after the infective episode. Epilepsy after meningitis is more likely if there is persistent neurological deficit (other than sensineural hearing loss). In developing countries, meningitis caused by Myco-bacterium tuberculosis frequently leads to subsequent seizure disorder. Cerebral abscesses from any cause can lead to refractory epilepsy, particularly if affecting the frontal lobe.

Immunisation
Concern about a link between increased seizure frequency and pertussis vaccine was common in the U.K. in the 1970s. A recent study of 368,000 children in the U.S.A. found it reassuring that if there is any risk associated with the [DPT] vaccine, its absolute magnitude is so low that it can not be detected in a study of that size (Gale et al., 1994).

Cerebrovascular Disease
Cerebrovascular disease is a common cause of epilepsy in people over the age of 60 years. In acute strokes, seizures can accompany a stroke (Hopkins, 1995). Strokes are very rare in children and they are usually accompanied by hemiparesis or weakness down one side of the body. The diagnosis can be confirmed by a CAT scan or an MRI brain scan (McMenamin and O'Connor Bird, 1997).

Degenerative Cerebral Disease
Seizures are more common in patients with Alzheimer's disease, Huntington's Chorea and occasionally in prion protein diseases (Hopkins, 1995).

Brain Malformations
A child with a brain malformation is very likely to be intellectually impaired and have other symptoms as well as epilepsy. The diagnosis can be confirmed by a CAT scan or an MRI brain scan (Mc Menamin and O'Connor Bird, 1997).

Cerebral Tumors
In the National General Practice Study of Epilepsy, Sander et al. (1990) reported that 6% of newly diagnosed patients with epilepsy were found to have a tumour. Features suggestive of a cerebral tumour are headaches, development of focal signs, postictal paresis, change in character of the epilepsy, status epilepticus or resistance to drug therapy (Hopkins, 1995).

Toxic Causes
Toxic causes include heavy metals, e.g., lead (particularly in children), or alcohol. Many drugs lower seizure threshold (Hopkins, 1995).

Metabolic Causes
These include: severe renal failure, hypoxia, over-hydration, hypoglycaemia, hyperglycaemia, low or high calcium levels, hypomagnesaemia, low pyridoxine and inborn errors of metabolism in children (Hopkins, 1995).

Chromosomal Abnormalities
These are usually associated with intellectual disability, abnormal physical features, unusual facial features and malformations of other organs of the body. Diagnosis is usually obvious but chromosomal studies, performed on white blood cells or skin cells are usually done (McMenamin and O'Connor Bird, 1997).

Rare Metabolic Disorders
Rare metabolic disorders associated with regression in development, failure to thrive, recurrent vomiting and other symptoms may also be associated with epilepsy (McMenamin and O'Connor Bird, 1997).

Known Causes of Seizures
Local Causes:
- Congenital, e.g. tuberose sclerosis
- Traumatic, e.g. perinatal*, head injury*, surgical.
- Inflammatory, e.g. meningitis*, acute and subacute encephalitis, neurosyphilis
- Neoplastic, e.g. tumour*, abscess, hematoma, aneurysm, angioma
- Degenerative, e.g. Alzheimers, Picks, lipidoses, thrombosis, hypertension, cerebrovascular disease*

General Causes
- Exogenous poisons, e.g. alcohol*, drugs* (e.g. theophyllines), drug withdrawal (e.g. anticonvulsants)
- Anoxia, e.g. respiratory failure, cardiac arrest
- Disordered metabolism, e.g. hypoglycemia*, hypocalcaemia, uraemia*, hepatic | encephalopathy

*Denotes commonest causes   (O'Connor et al., 1992)

1.7 TRIGGERS

For most people there is no single factor that is known to trigger epileptic seizures. The cause of seizures in one person will have no effect on another, and sometimes it is not even possible to detect any one factor responsible for the seizures of an individual. However, some people with epilepsy can identify factors that trigger seizures.

In their information booklet, Epilepsy, Questions and Answers (1992), Brainwave, the Irish Epilepsy Association state that about 5% of people who have epilepsy are photosensitive and may have a seizure in response to flickering lights, such as strobe lights or even the flicker of sunlight through trees. Other known precipitating factors are lack of sleep, exhaustion, lack of food, anxiety, boredom, emotional stress, excess alcohol, abrupt cessation of anti-epileptic medication and, in photosensitive epilepsy particularly, shimmering or very regular light patterns. The causes of seizures in some people are very complex and may be related to body metabolism and chemical changes. For instance, it is recognised that many women with epilepsy are more at risk of seizures either during, or immediately before menstruation (McGovern, 1985).

Precipitating factors such as physical and mental overstrain, intense fear, pain or rage may trigger seizures in a predisposed child with any kind of epilepsy. Worry and anxiety over problems at school and at home, such as the prospect of a move to a new school or a new class, or parental illness often act in the same way. Minor medical manipulations, such as blood tests, dental treatment or minor surgical operations, may also trigger a seizure. It is rare for children to have fits during examinations but a child is liable to have a seizure when exposed to an environment with which he cannot cope (Egg-Olofsson, 1985).

1.8 EPIDEMIOLOGY

1.8.1 Introduction

Epilepsy is the most common serious neurological condition, with a prevalence rate 10-fold higher than that of multiple sclerosis and 100-fold higher than that of motor neurone disease (Brodie et al. 1997). The study of the epidemiology of epilepsy is beset with problems for many reasons. O'Donohue (1994) refers to the fact that if epilepsy is associated with a social stigma, the presence of seizures may be denied and the disease remains hidden. The lack of a uniformly accepted definition and classification for epilepsy makes it difficult to compare the results of different epidemiological investigations. The study of epilepsy is further complicated by the fact that one is dealing with a symptom complex which may be a manifestation of a large number of diverse disease entities, each with a different cause, some of which are known and some unknown. The definition of what constitutes epilepsy also varies, with some investigators including single, isolated seizures or febrile convulsions.

1.8.2 Incidence

The incidence of epilepsy in most developed countries is 50-70 cases per 100,000 persons per year. There are no marked differences among different European countries or regions.

Incidence varies greatly with age, with high rates in early childhood, decreasing to low levels in early adult life, but with a second peak in people aged more than 65 years. Most studies suggest slight excess in males. In recent years, the absolute numbers of affected children has decreased and the number of elderly people with epilepsy has sharply increased (Brodie et al. 1997).

1.8.3 Prevalence

Prevalence rates show the number of individuals with active epilepsy at a given time. According to Brodie et al. (1997), the prevalence of epilepsy is 5-10 cases per 1,000 population. This figure excludes both febrile convulsions, which occur in 5% of children, and single seizures. No marked differences exist among different European countries or regions. The lifetime prevalence is 5%. Therefore, as many as one in 20 of the population will experience a seizure at some time in their lives.

According to Sidenvall (1990), persons with epilepsy should have recurrent, non-provoked epileptic seizures within the past one, three or five years, or be on prophylactic medication. Figures for prevalence rates vary from 1.5 to 33.7 per 1000 (Tsuboi, 1984) but more studies cluster between 3 and 6 per 1,000 (Hauser, 1978).

The variation in prevalence figures may be due to differences in definition, intensity of case selection, or a true difference between populations. In a review of case selection methods for recurrent afebrile seizures in Japan, Tsuboi (1984) found that data collected by questionnaire gave a mean prevalence rate of 14/1000, by records from general practitioners and medical record reviews 6/1000 and by clinical examination 12/1000.

There is also the risk that persons with epilepsy will never seek medical advice. In a field study of 15,000 Warsaw residents (Zielinski, 1974) one-third of the group with epilepsy (defined as more than two afebrile seizures) were on anti-epileptic drugs and one-third had had treatment earlier. Of those with epilepsy, 26% had never been diagnosed. This group often had partial seizures or generalised absence seizures.

Exact measures of prevalence are difficult to establish (Sander and Shorvon, 1987), but the proportion of the population receiving treatment for epilepsy is about 0.5%, with a lifetime incidence of 2% (Goodridge and Shorvon, 1983). In a list of 2,000 patients one would expect to find four children and seven adults with active epilepsy (that is, either on treatment or getting seizures off treatment) and 35 patients who have had epilepsy at some stage in their life and are now in remission (Royal College of General Practitioners, London, 1992).

For the Scandinavian countries there is a variation in prevalence from 12.7/1000 in Denmark to 2.3 or 3.5/1000 in Northern Norway, all ages included (Sidenvall, 1990). Studies on British populations, which may be closer to the Irish situation, indicate a prevalence rate of 11/1000 of children under the age of 14 experiencing active epilepsy. Further research suggests that 31-65% of these cases have primary generalised epilepsy, while 34-43% have partial epilepsy (Kurtz, 1983). It is estimated that at least one in every 200 people has some form of epilepsy. In their information booklet, Your Guide to Epilepsy, (1998). Brainwave, the Irish Epilepsy Association, state that this means that as many as 20,000 people in Ireland could be affected by epilepsy.

1.9 SUMMARY
This chapter has examined the nature of epilepsy; definitions, classifications, types of seizures and aetiology. The definitions which are applied to the condition by various professionals and organisations, such as WHO and the Irish and British Epilepsy Associations, were outlined. Classifications of seizures, as determined by the International League Against Epilepsy, were identified. The varying types of seizures, whether generalised or partial, were also examined. The many causes of the condition, such as genetic and hereditary, prenatal and perinatal, were considered under aetiology. Epidemiology, including prevalence and incidence, were also discussed.

At present, it appears that there is no co-ordinated body of data available in any Irish Governmental Department or Health Board concerning such basic information as the number of people with epilepsy in the State. Based on studies on British populations, Brainwave, the Irish Epilepsy Association estimate that the likely prevalence rate of epilepsy in Ireland is 1 in 200 or 20,000 people. The lack of an established and co-ordinated incidence and prevalence rate of epilepsy among the Irish adult and child population makes it difficult to establish their medical and educational needs.

CHAPTER TWO

HISTORICAL CONCEPTIONS OF EPILEPSY

2.1   INTRODUCTION

From early times, epilepsy has been considered 'a special disease, a weird illness and a strange malady' (LeBrun, 1992). The behavioural manifestations of epilepsy have always aroused great interest and controversy, and there is little doubt that its historical legacy has shaped public attitudes to epilepsy. This historical legacy has been reviewed in the classic work of Temkin (1994). Many names have been used to describe the condition over the centuries, and these reflect some fundamental aspects of the beliefs and prejudices that were, or still are, entertained concerning the condition. There are few other illnesses whose many names tell so much about past prejudices and misconceptions.

The various names ascribed to the condition over the centuries are reviewed in this chapter. The beliefs surrounding the practice of adopting a patron saint to protect against the supposed evils of epilepsy in various countries are examined. Developments in the medical field of epilepsy during the nineteenth and twentieth centuries are traced, and legislation relating to issues such as marriage, adoption or immigration for persons with epilepsy is summarised.

2.2   THE DISEASE OF MANY NAMES
2.2.1 Sacred or Holy Disease

The ancient Greeks believed that epilepsy was the most sacred and psychological of all diseases and was the result of the invasion of the body by a god. It was believed that only a god could deprive a sane and healthy man of his senses, throw him to the ground, convulse him and then rapidly restore him to his former self. Hence the title 'On the Sacred Disease' which Hippocrates, a Greek physician who lived around 450 BC, gave to the book in which he dealt with epilepsy. Hippocrates, the father of medicine, argued against the prevalent belief that epilepsy was divinely inspired, and claimed that epilepsy was no more divine or sacred than any other disease. He claimed that, like all diseases, it had a natural cause and was hereditary, with its cause residing in the brain, a brain 'overflowing with a superfluity of phlegm, one of the four humours or body fluids' (Temkin, 1994). For thousands of years people thought that the body contained four different liquids - blood, black and red gall, and phlegm. The cause of epilepsy, they believed, was a build-up of phlegm in the arteries leading to the head, resulting in the air supply being cut off. It was believed that blood circulated in the veins only, while the arteries carried air. The sight of foam around the mouth of a person having a fit was taken as proof of the accumulation of phlegm. Galen, a physician who lived in the 1st Century AD, believed that phlegm built up in an arm or leg and from there spread to the rest of the body. This explained why convulsions started in an arm or leg and then spread to the rest of the body. As treatment, the tourniquet was used. Amputation was also employed, as it was thought to stop the spread of the damaging substances, a method of treatment, which, in the case of snakebite, was known to be successful. If the seizures did not have a localized start, more drastic methods were used to remove the phlegm, which by then was thought to have reached the head. This was done by trephinning, where a triangular hole was chiselled out of the skull to create a 'drain'. These holes were often made at the rear of the skull, as it was thought that phlegm sank to the bottom at the back of the head (Dam and Gram, 1986). Many physicians also recommended that tablets could solve all the problems of any curable epilepsy. These tablets were to be made from substances such as the rib of the left side of a man who had been hanged or beheaded, and given to the patient, with water, every morning for a month.

Unfortunately, the Hippocratic view of epilepsy being a natural disorder was not widely accepted, and for centuries the disease continued to be regarded as a sickness of supernatural origin. The Romans called it morbus sacer, morbus divinus or lues deifica, i.e. the sacred disease or the divine plague. In France it was referred to as the mal sacre, mal (de) sainct, mal divin or haut mal. The Germans spoke of heilige Krankheit, heiliges Weh (sacred disease) or das Hochste (the supreme). In the dialect of Mecklenburg the disease used to be called dat hillig (the holy disease) (Lebrun, 1992).

In ancient Rome, if a person had a seizure during a comitia, i.e. an assembly of the people, the assembly had to be dispersed, because the occurrence of the seizure was considered to be an ominous sign. Epilepsy, therefore, was often called morbus comitialis. The adjective comitial is still used in French medical jargon to refer to epilepsy.

Although the Greeks ascribed epilepsy to divine intervention, later opinion held that demons, rather than gods, were responsible. In Greek epileptos meant not only epileptic but also controlled by a spirit. Epilepsy was also called le mauvais mal or la male passion (the wicked disease) in French, and boses Wesen (wicked spirit) in German (Lebrun, 1992).

This belief gained ascendancy by the time of the Christian gospel writers, and is alluded to in the miracle recounting how Jesus cured a boy with epilepsy by exorcising him. In the Gospel account of St. Mark (Ch. 9: 17-29), a man whose son was suffering from fits came to Jesus saying, "Teacher, I brought my son to you, because he has an evil spirit in him and cannot talk. Whenever the spirit attacks him, it throws him to the ground, and he foams at the mouth, grits his teeth, and becomes stiff all over." When Jesus asked how long he had been like that, the father said, "Ever since he was a child. Many times the evil spirit has tried to kill him by throwing him in the fire and into water." When Jesus noticed that the crowd was closing in on them, he rebuked the spirit, saying to him, "Deaf and dumb spirit, I order you to come out of the boy and never go into him again." The spirit screamed, threw the boy into a bad fit, and came out. The boy looked like a corpse, and everyone said, "He is dead!" but Jesus took the boy by the hand and helped him to rise, and he stood up" (Good News Bible, Today's English Version, 1976).

It must be noted that neither Jesus nor the child's father refers to the term epilepsy. However, in the gospel according to St. Matthew, (Ch.17: 14-20), the boy's father said to Jesus, "Sir, have mercy on my son! He is an epileptic and has such terrible fits that he often falls in the fire or into water" (Good News Bible, Today's English Version, 1976). These passages from scripture give a clear description of a grand mal epileptic attack and illustrate the prevailing belief of the child with epilepsy suffering from demonical possession.

In ancient Egypt, people with epilepsy were advised to eat the excrement of donkeys diluted in wine. This was meant to sicken the demon inside and cause him to leave the sufferer's body. In some places in India, a red-hot iron was applied to the foreheads of persons with epilepsy to drive out the evil spirit (Lebrun, 1992).

2.2.2 Lunar Disease
The mythology surrounding epilepsy also included a supposed link between epilepsy and lunacy, and the idea that it could be caused by heavenly bodies and the influence of the cycle of the moon. It was therefore also called morbus lunaticus or morbus astralis in Latin, mal lunatique in French, and maanziekte (moon sickness) in Dutch. In Greek, seleniakos, an adjective derived from selene (moon), meant epileptic. In Anglo-Saxon countries, people with epilepsy were often said to be 'moonstruck' (Lebrun 1992). Hence, the word 'lunatic' was first applied to sufferers of epilepsy, while mad people were 'maniacs' whose madness was as a result of invasion of the body by devils or evil spirits, not gods. However, over time the distinction became blurred and people with epilepsy were regarded as both lunatic and maniac! (Reynolds, 1989).

In the 19th century, a beverage supposed to be efficacious against epilepsy was given twice a year to sufferers in Tain-L'Hermitage on the River Rhone in France. The drug, which was prepared with white cheese-rennet, was called 'le grand remede' (the great remedy), and had to be taken when the moon was full. Many sufferers who came to drink the remedy wore masks to hide their identity. Nowadays, a potion is still sold in and around Tain-L'Hermitage under the name of 'Grand Remede de l'Hermitage', but it contains more bromide than cheese-rennet (Lebrun, 1992).

Even Galen, although he was a biologist who believed that the immediate causes of epilepsy were 'humoral' or 'toxic', held that the moon regulated the occasions of the fits, which return when the moon is full (Hill, 1981). The association of epilepsy with the moon, and more specifically with the moon cycles, may in part be due to the fact that for some women with epilepsy, seizures only occur, or increase in frequency, during menstrual periods.

2.2.3 Infamous Disease
People with epilepsy were often debarred from a number of positions or privileges, including the priesthood. In early Christian times, people with epilepsy were refused Holy Communion. In many places, the sale of a slave was void if the slave turned out to have epilepsy. However, at times epilepsy was associated with supernatural gifts. People with epilepsy were regarded as soothsayers or prophets, and attacks were deemed to be of the same nature as moments of artistic inspiration (Lebrun, 1992).

2.2.4 Contagious Disease
Epilepsy was considered contagious and the person with epilepsy was regarded as unclean. It was thought that whoever touched them might become prey to the demons. As a preventive measure, it was a common Roman custom to spit at people with the illness in order to repel 'evil spirits' and throw back contagion and infection. For this reason, another name for the disease was morbus insputatus (the disease you spit at) in Latin. The Romans used to plant a nail where a person with epilepsy had fallen in order to prevent the disease from propagating (Lebrun, 1992).

For the epilepsy sufferer, life was indeed miserable and such a person was subject to extreme degradation. To the general public he was merely an object of horror and disgust. The Roman author, Apuleius, when writing about a slave boy, Thallus, said that his fellow slaves would have nothing to do with him because of his epilepsy:

> "Nobody dares to eat with him from the same dish or drink from
> the same cup lest he contaminate the family" (Rogan, 1980).

It was also thought for a time that epilepsy was an infectious disease, caused by various poisons or toxins which could attack the body from the outside. Seizures were regarded as the body's attempt to get rid of these poisonous substances, in exactly the same way as it was believed that hiccups were the stomach's attempt to empty itself of damaging food. The presumption of the illness' infectious nature sometimes gave rise to a marked social discrimination against the sufferers. The illness was often seen as a form of a curse, something one wished on one's worst enemies. Epilepsy was also among the plagues Martin Luther called down on the Catholic Church! (Dam and Gram, 1986).

People with epilepsy were often confined with the insane. Esquirol, a 19th century physician, pleaded for the establishment of special divisions for people with epilepsy. He believed, as many others did, that the mere sight of an epileptic attack might make a healthy person develop epilepsy. Since the mentally deranged were more impressionable than healthy people, the likelihood of their developing epilepsy after witnessing a seizure was even greater. Accordingly, it was considered that people with epilepsy should be confined to minimise the danger to other patients. In the second half of the 19th century, the inhabitants of Tain-L'Hermitage campaigned for the closing down of the hospital for people with epilepsy in the town because they were afraid of being contaminated by the patients (Lebrun, 1992).

2.2.5 Hereditary Disease
Epilepsy was also believed to be hereditary. In many countries people with epilepsy were not allowed to marry. In some parts of India a marriage can still be made void if it appears that one of the partners had epilepsy before marriage, but concealed the fact (Lebrun, 1992).

2.2.6 Falling Sickness
The disease was also called falling sickness, falling ill or falling evil. In French, epilepsy was also called mal de terre, i.e. ground or earth disease, possibly because the sufferers fall to the ground (Lebrun, 1992).

2.2.7 Dreadful Disease
Epilepsy was a dreaded disease and therefore, even its name was taboo in many countries. Euphemisms, which had a propitious function, were often used. The French spoke of the beau mal (the good disease) or simply le mal (the disease). Epilepsy was considered to be a serious handicap, hence its Latin names of morbus sonticus (severe illness) and morbus maior (great

disease). The French spoke of grande maladie, grand mal or gros mal (fateful disease) and the Germans of schwere (great predicament) (Lebrun, 1992).

Epilepsy was also considered to be a shameful disease, and the unfortunate person who felt an attack coming on often rushed home or to a deserted place where he covered his head. To the ancients, the epileptic was an object of horror and disgust, and throughout the ages those afflicted have been viewed with anxiety and fear. O'Donohue (1994) believes that no other illness has set individuals apart so far, so often and for so long, and he contends that some of these attitudes persist to the present day.

2.2.8 Epilepsy
The word epilepsy is derived from the Greek verb epilambanein, which means 'to take hold of', 'to seize' or 'to attack'. The image survives in the English word seizure. An epileptic attack may also be called an ictus. This word originally meant a blow or a stroke. The derived adjectives post-ictal and interictal are often used to refer to behaviours during, after or between seizures.

The word aura, which is similar to the word air, means breeze or zephyr. It is often used to refer to the premonitory symptom(s) of a seizure, because the Greek physician Galen once heard a boy with epilepsy liken the sensation that he felt before an attack to a cold breeze blowing on a part of his body. The word aura nowadays denotes any sensation that the patient perceives just prior to an attack and which is recognised as a forerunner to a seizure (Lebrun, 1992). From the time of Hippocrates physicians wrote about 'convulsions', particularly with reference to children, without clearly defining the meaning of the term and its relationship to epilepsy. There was awareness in medical writing that convulsions in early childhood might have a different prognostic significance from epileptic seizures in older persons, but for a long time the terminology remained confused. Attitudes to children with epilepsy were unenlightened and often cruel until well into the nineteenth century, and children frequently suffered the general fate of epileptics in being confined with insane persons (O'Donohue, 1994).

2.3 SAINTS AGAINST THE DISEASE
With the spread of Christianity, saints were adopted as the patrons of those afflicted with what was then called the 'falling sickness'. St. Valentine was considered patron saint of the epileptics, and epilepsy was often called mal St.Valentin (St.Valentine's disease) in French. The Germans used St. Veltinskrankheit, St. Veltinsplage (St. Valentine's plague) or St.Veltinsarbeit (St.Valentine's toil). In Dutch, sintvelten became a synonym for epilepsy, as did Sankt Veltin in German. One could curse another with the words "Ich wolt dasz er Sanct Veltin het!" (I wish he had St. Valentine, i.e. epilepsy).

St. Lupus was a protector against epilepsy and the disease was sometimes called morbus St. Lupi or morbus Beati Lupi in Latin, and mal (de) Saint Loup or Mal Saint Leu in French. Legend has it that someone misbehaved at the burial of this saint and was stricken with epilepsy, but eventually repented and was cured.

St. John was another saint often invoked against the disease, which was often called mal Saint Jean in French and St. Janseuvel or St. Jansplaag in Dutch. It is not clear whether the patron was St. John the Baptist or St. John the Evangelist, nor why precisely he was invoked against epilepsy.

In Germanic countries, St. Cornelius was the saint called upon to assist in cases of epilepsy or to protect one from the disease. In Belgium, until recently, children were often given four names at birth. The fourth name was frequently Cornelius or its feminine form, Cornelia. By giving their child the name of the saint, parents sought to protect it from epilepsy (Lebrun, 1992).

2.4 EPILEPSY DURING THE NINETEENTH CENTURY
The process of distinguishing epilepsy from madness began in the nineteenth century and was linked with the development of neurology. It was the discoveries of neurology which began to challenge these deeply entrenched concepts of demoniac possession as a cause for epilepsy, since the new neurologists encountered much epilepsy without mental illness in their private practice. In 1859, the first neurological hospital in the world, the National Hospital for the Paralysed and Epileptic, was opened in London. Among its brilliant staff were Russell Reynolds (1828 -1896),

William Gowers (1845 -1915) and John Hughlings Jackson (1834 -1911). In the latter half of the nineteenth century, views about epilepsy were radically changed by Jackson (1873), who suggested that the word should be redefined in neurophysiological rather than clinical terms. It was Jackson who gave the first scientifically accurate definition of epilepsy, which is still accepted as valid: 'Epilepsy is the name for occasional, sudden, excessive, rapid and local discharges of nerve tissue' (Hill, 1981).

This was the first neuronal theory of epilepsy, and it is from this that the modern epileptologists have defined and redefined the various forms of clinical epilepsy. The discovery of the electroencephalogram (EEG) by Hans Berger in 1929 and his observations on the neurological characteristics of epilepsy further facilitated the separation of epilepsy from other conditions and offered visual proof of Hughlings Jackson's theories (O'Donohue, 1994).

2.5   EPILEPSY DURING THE TWENTIETH CENTURY

At the beginning of this century, psychiatric views about the nature of epilepsy still dominated the literature. Geurrant et al. (1962) describes three new phases of evolution in thinking since then. In the early part of this century the concept of the "epileptic character" held sway. According to this view the epileptic patient could be identified by certain personality traits, mostly of an antisocial nature. However, from the studies of William Lennox in the 1930s and the 1940s, it became increasingly more widely accepted that most patients with epilepsy had normal mental states. The culmination of this process has been that, over the last thirty years, the diagnosis of epilepsy has finally been removed from national and international classifications of psychiatric illness (Hill, 1981). Other more recent contributions to the understanding of epilepsy have been those of Lennox and Lennox (1960), Guerrant et al. (1962), Hill (1981) and Berrios (1984).

2.6   LAWS RELATING TO EPILEPSY

Specific laws regarding the marriage of people with epilepsy, the validity of their court testimony and rights of owners of slaves with epilepsy may be found as far back as 2000 BC in the Babylonian Law of Hammurabbi. A clause in the law said that a slave could only be sold if the purchaser was given a money-back guarantee should bennu (epilepsy) appear within the month after the purchase (Temkin, 1994).

As recently as 1939, a law was enacted in North Carolina to control the marriage of people with epilepsy. The first modern anti-marriage laws for those with epilepsy were probably those devised in Sweden beginning in 1757 (Gunn, 1981). In the United States seventeen states prohibited persons with epilepsy from marrying, and it was only as recently as 1980 that the last state repealed its laws forbidding marriage to people with epilepsy (McLin and de Boer, 1995). The laws varied in type, some making marriages void, others imposing penal sanctions or fines or even imprisonment of up to three years should a person with epilepsy marry. The situation was no better in other countries. In the United Kingdom, a law prohibiting people with epilepsy from marrying was not repealed until 1970. In some parts of the world epilepsy is still commonly viewed as a reason for annulment of marriage (McLin and de Boer, 1995).

Twenty-eight of the U.S. states have also had, at some time, some form of sterilisation law allowing those with epilepsy to be sterilised either by consent, or in some states, by court order (Gunn, 1981). In 1956, eighteen states still had statutes that allowed eugenic sterilisation of people with epilepsy (McLin and de Boer, 1995).

Gunn (1981) states that although no western country actually uses any of these statutes now, epilepsy is still a bar to immigration to some countries. The Australian Embassy only removed their direct prohibition on epilepsy ten years ago. Following inquiries to the Australian Immigration Authorities regarding visa requirements, the researcher was informed (Appendix 1) that an application cannot be refused on medical grounds if the applicant who has epilepsy can show that it is well-controlled and that he or she does not make excessive use of medical services and holds a job and driving licence! It might therefore be inferred that these regulations may still be exclusionary for certain persons with epilepsy, as, given the nature of many types of seizures, many people with epilepsy might often find it very difficult to be confident that their epilepsy is controlled and consequently, may not have a driving licence. Applicants are undoubtedly assessed on their need for care and treatment, and it was stated that visas might certainly be refused if it is felt that significant care and treatment are required. Epilepsy usually does require medication and treatment, so this constitutes another basis on which a visa may be refused.

Policies on adoption were another area where people with epilepsy were discriminated against. In some areas of the United States, an adoption could be annulled if the child later developed epilepsy. Until 1978, Arkansas and Missouri allowed adoptions to be annulled if the child developed epilepsy within five years. In Europe there is no legislation concerning epilepsy and adoption. In a few cases, problems in the adoption of children with epilepsy have been reported, but it is not known whether the epilepsy itself played a significant role in those decisions. It is clear, however, that when an adoption was denied or annulled because of a diagnosis of epilepsy in either parent or child, the unequivocal public message was that people with epilepsy might be 'damaged goods' (McLin and de Boer, 1995).

Another area from which people with epilepsy were debarred was ordination. This is based on the Code of Canon Law (1983), Canon 1041 No. 1, which excludes from the priesthood any one '.. who suffers from any form of insanity, or from any other psychological infirmity, because of which he is, after experts have been consulted, judged incapable of being able to fulfil the ministry' (Appendix 2). That this exclusion also relates to epilepsy might be inferred from the recent case of a twenty-eight year old man who had been seizure-free while studying in the priesthood for the first two years. When he did experience a seizure he was told that he would not be ordained to the priesthood and that he ".. should leave of his own accord rather than be asked to leave, which would look bad on any future reference"(Clancy, 1998). Therefore, it would appear that the Roman Catholic Church retains a certain discretion to exclude a person with epilepsy from ordination under Canon 104 No. 1, 'on medical advice given to the Bishop'.

While this canon was removed from the Ecclesiastical Law (1873) governing the Church of Ireland after the Reformation, it was replaced by an ordnance giving absolute discretion to the Church of Ireland bishops as to whom they shall or shall not ordain (Appendix 2). It is therefore unclear whether epilepsy constitutes grounds for exclusion for ordination in the Church of Ireland.

Prejudices about epilepsy were similarly reinforced by practices related to institutionalisation. As recently as 1956, four States in the U.S. permitted a person to be institutionalised based solely on a diagnosis of epilepsy with uncontrolled seizures (McLin and de Boer, 1995). In Europe, special centres for those with epilepsy have existed for more than a century. In Ireland, two such 'colonies' existed: Moore Abbey in Monasterevin, Co. Kildare and St. John of Gods' in Mulhuddart, Co.Dublin. In a telephone conversation with a nun in Moore Abbey, the researcher was told how many of the people in these institutions were sent there solely on the basis of their epilepsy, in order to hide them from the outside world. This was due to public ignorance and misunderstanding about the condition. However, Sr. X stated that this situation has gradually changed as a result of better control of seizures with improved medication. McLin and de Boer (1995) believe that changing attitudes and the high cost of institutional care have closed many such centres, or caused others to redirect their efforts to more appropriate therapeutic or rehabilitative care.

2.7 SUMMARY

This chapter explored some of the more prevalent historical conceptions of epilepsy. The various names that were given to epilepsy through the centuries were outlined, giving an overview of the ideas and prejudices that were entertained about the disease. They vividly recount the different, usually prejudicial ways in which the illness was perceived.

The process of distinguishing epilepsy from a demonic disease can be linked to the development of neurology and the discovery of the electroencephalogram (EEG) in the 19th century. From the studies of William Lennox in the 1930s and 1940s, it became more widely accepted that the concept of the "epileptic personality" was unacceptable. The culmination of this process was the removal of epilepsy from the international classifications of psychiatric illnesses.

Nevertheless, not all prejudices concerning epilepsy have been eradicated, as is shown in practices relating to areas such as ordination and immigration. Stances by immigration and religious authorities only serve to reinforce existing prejudices. It is not until such issues are addressed that negative attitudes to epilepsy will change.

CHAPTER THREE

ATTITUDES TOWARDS AND BELIEFS ABOUT EPILEPSY

3.1   INTRODUCTION

Among the many illnesses and handicaps that exist, epilepsy has always been regarded with some awe and fear (Dinnage, 1986). In view of the ancient beliefs and myths that have been associated with epilepsy over the centuries, it is not surprising to find that it can still carry a stigma. Although both attitudes towards, and treatment of, people with epilepsy have changed tremendously over the past centuries, de Boer (1995) believes that not all problems have been solved. She states that in almost every country prejudice still exists and strange beliefs influence society's attitudes. Having epilepsy, even today, sometimes presents insurmountable problems.

According to Chung et al. (1995), persons with epilepsy frequently experience psychosocial difficulties in terms of interpersonal relationships and jobs. These problems are not always related to the severity of the seizure disorder, but instead relate to discrimination or misconceptions, mainly due to beliefs that persons with epilepsy are physically disabled, mentally retarded or emotionally disturbed.

Gordon and Sillanpaa (1997) also stress how the attitude of others towards a person who has epileptic seizures is a factor of great importance in that person's life. This applies at all ages but presents particular problems in childhood (Gordon and Sillanpaa, 1997; de Boer, 1995). According to Gordon and Sillanpaa (1997), mainstream schools may be able to cope with most children with disabilities if the disability is not too severe, but not if they also have epilepsy. They feel that this is mainly due to people's attitudes, but also to lack of resources.

This chapter looks at the issue of stigma as it applies to epilepsy. It considers public perceptions of people with epilepsy, and the factors that contribute to these attitudes.

3.2   THE STIGMA OF EPILEPSY

Dell (1986) defines stigma as the relation "between the differentness of an individual and the devaluation society places on that particular differentness". Epilepsy is still shrouded in misinformation and misbelief. For many people with epilepsy, coping with the stigma surrounding the disorder is more difficult than living with any limitations imposed by the seizures themselves or by their treatment (Commission for the Control of Epilepsy and its Consequences, 1978).

According to Baker et al. (1997) some other chronic conditions are also stigmatising, but epilepsy, for reasons rooted deep in its history, is a stigmatising condition par excellence. Due to uncertainty concerning its clinical origins and its social connotations, the impact of epilepsy on a person's quality of life can be significant. Baker et al. (1997), in a survey of quality of life of people with epilepsy in 15 countries in Europe, reported that over half of all respondents (n=2,525) felt stigmatised by their epilepsy. In a study of patient perceptions of their condition, Hayden et al. (1992) found that 44% (n=228) of the respondents believed that others, but not everyone whom they came into contact with, saw them as being different. When asked to mention a matter which concerned them most about their epilepsy, 10% (n=52) said they were worried about the stigma of epilepsy and the related social implications of the condition. Other issues of concern included public ignorance about epilepsy, and worries about employment and career matters. Forty-six per cent (n=238) of respondents perceived employment as one of their major problems.

McLin and de Boer (1995) believe that because people with epilepsy have so often internalised society's devaluation of them, they have not felt empowered to change the situation. Negative stereotypes of persons with epilepsy have been so ingrained in the collective belief system that they have become an accepted part of many people's concept of the disorder. At an awareness day held by Brainwave, the Irish Epilepsy Association, in September 1998, the researcher noted that many (n=30) of the young people attending one of the workshops commented that they had experienced discrimination because of their epilepsy. One girl said that epilepsy was "..a catching disease that made people keep away from you." She reported that she had been badly treated by the girls in her school, and that only two girls were friendly to her. She commented that one of these girls' fathers was a doctor and her brother was autistic, so this other girl knew what she was going through. This experience also illustrates how knowledge of a condition can help people be more understanding and accepting.

However, Scrambler and Hopkins (1990) argue that the discrimination that people with epilepsy perceive may be as important a factor as the actual discrimination of others, - "felt stigma" as opposed to "enacted stigma." Among people who develop epilepsy in later life, the fear of seizures may be greater than the fear of the stigma attached to the diagnosis but in time other psychosocial problems will almost certainly arise (Chaplin et al. 1992).

Jacoby and Chadwick (1992) believe that the adjustment of those with epilepsy to their disability is fundamental to their well being, and if this adjustment is well managed, it can often help to remove the feeling of stigma. However, Austin et al. (1994) warn that when epilepsy is associated with evidence of brain damage, adaptation is likely to be impeded.

Gordon and Sillanpaa (1997) also argue that if an individual believes that their condition caries a stigma, others will almost certainly agree. They believe that one predictor of self-acceptance is how those with epilepsy feel about other people with disabilities. Ingwell et al. (1967) reported that, in general, people with epilepsy have negative attitudes towards others with disabilities, even though such negative attitudes may be less in evidence than those held by healthy individuals.

3.3   PUBLIC PERCEPTIONS OF EPILEPSY

Chung et al. (1995) states that establishing the degree of awareness and understanding of epilepsy in a society is a necessary initial step in eliminating discrimination against persons with epilepsy. There have been a number of international studies and surveys on public awareness and attitudes to people with epilepsy. Among the most pessimistic study is that by Bagley (1972), who found that a large proportion of the respondents opposed the employment of people with epilepsy, and that a sample of teenagers ranked those with epilepsy below those with cerebral palsy and mental retardation on questions relating to their suitability for work, marriage and housing. As these opinions were more extreme than those found by other researchers, these findings may have been due to the number of young and inexperienced people in the sample. Tringo's (1970) subjects in the U.S.A. also rated epilepsy very poorly in a hierarchy of physical and mental handicaps, but again the subjects were secondary school and college students. A campaign by Sands and Zalkind (1972) in the U.S.A., to educate employers about epilepsy, was found to have no effects on negative attitudes towards employing persons with epilepsy. These studies are not encouraging but they were conducted in the 1970s. The following surveys, however, report that there is evidence that attitudes to epilepsy may be becoming more informed.

Iivanainen et al. (1980), in a study of 2,272 people in Finland, reported that 95% (n=2,158) of the respondents had heard of epilepsy, 49% (n=1,113) knew someone with epilepsy and 45% (n=1,022) had witnessed a seizure taking place. These percentages were surprisingly high. Attitudes towards children with epilepsy were more charitable than those towards adults, and familiarity with someone having seizures was the most important factor in the development of enlightened attitudes to those with epilepsy. The study was repeated in 1983 (Uutela and Sillanpaa, 1985) and showed a general improvement in attitudes towards people with epilepsy. It was noted that attitudes were more positive in urban than in rural areas and more positive towards children than towards adults. These changes had taken place as a result of a nationwide campaign for more public knowledge about, and more enlightened attitudes towards, epilepsy. Public knowledge about epilepsy was found to have increased more than an enlightenment of attitudes (Uutela and Sillanpaa, 1985).

Jenson and Dam (1992) conducted a survey of 1,500 people in Denmark aged over 15 years. Of the 69% (n=1,035) who responded, 97% (n=1,004) had heard or read about epilepsy. The survey found that attitudes in Denmark towards people with epilepsy were generally favourable but, 7% (n=105) had objections to social contact between their children and people with the condition, suggesting that there has been no startling changes in attitude in recent years. Jenson and Dam

(1992) stress that the general population needs more information about epilepsy. They advocate continuous and effective campaigns to improve public knowledge and attitudes towards those with the condition, noting that medical students and general practitioners in Denmark also have insufficient knowledge of epilepsy.

Canger and Cornaggia (1985), in a survey of 1,043 (n=282) adults in Italy, found that 27% (n=282) of those surveyed did not know what epilepsy was. This was more evident among the elderly in the south of the country and in rural areas. Sixty-one per cent (n=636) knew someone who had epilepsy, and 52% (n=542) had seen a person having a seizure. When those who were familiar with epilepsy were asked if they would object to their child associating at school or at play with people who had seizures, 11% (n=70) replied that they would object. Although 70% (n=730) thought that those with epilepsy should be employed in normal occupations, 8% (n=83) thought that epilepsy was a form of insanity.

Finke (1980), having previously undertaken a survey of public attitudes towards epilepsy in Germany in 1967 and 1973, repeated the survey in 1978. While the size of the sample was not specified, 90% of those interviewed had heard of epilepsy and of these, 23% said they would object to their child playing with children who had epilepsy (in previous years these results had represented 37% and 27% of the sample respectively). The number of those who had thought that epilepsy was a form of insanity also decreased from 27% to 23%, and the percentage of those who objected to the employment of those with epilepsy fell from 31% to 20%. It was found that public bias in attitudes to epilepsy could be significantly associated with levels of education, increasing age and increasing urbanisation.

National surveys of this type have been carried out in the U.S.A. every five years since 1949. Of the 1,539 adults surveyed by Caveness and Gallup (1980), 95% (n=1,462) had heard or read about epilepsy. When those who knew about the condition were asked if they would object to their child playing with others who had epilepsy, 89% (n=1,301) said that they would not, a figure which had increased from 57% in 1949 There was a similar favourable trend from 59% to 92% amongst those who did not think epilepsy was a form of insanity. The percentage of respondents who agreed that persons with epilepsy should be employed rose from 45% to 79%. The most favourable opinions were generally found among the better-educated, better-employed, younger and urban members of the population. The improvement in attitudes over the years was particularly noticeable in the southern states. According to Baumann et al. (1995), contributory factors to this change in public opinion have been the development of more effective treatment to control seizures and the decrease in social stigma linked to epilepsy. However, in 1987, one in three Americans still believed that having epilepsy induced a negative bias towards those with the disorder and their families, and one in six continued to consider that epilepsy was a form of mental illness (LaMartina, 1989).

In a telephone survey conducted by Baumann et al. (1995), it was found that 24% (n=148) of Kentuckians predicted a deterioration in the classroom environment if a child with epilepsy was admitted. Forty-one per cent (n=253) said that the quality of their child's life would be lowered by the time he or she reached the age of 21 years if children with epilepsy were admitted to the class. The authors concluded that this finding confirms that in that particular area of the United States there is still significant prejudice towards those with epilepsy and that increase in public knowledge about the condition alone may not eliminate this.

Chung et al. (1995) conducted a survey of public awareness, understanding and attitudes towards epilepsy among 2,610 adults ranging in age from 15 to 91 years in Taiwan. Of the respondents, 87% (n=2,271) had read or heard about epilepsy, 70% (n=1,827) knew someone who had epilepsy and 56% (n=1,462) had seen someone having a seizure. Eighteen per cent (n=470) objected to having their children associate with people with epilepsy in school or at play. This negative attitude was associated with "older age, male gender and labour class". Seventy-two per cent (n=1,879) of the respondents would object to their children marrying a person with epilepsy, in contrast to 18% in the U.S study (Caveness and Gallup, 1980). Surprisingly this response was correlated with youth, married state and higher education. The authors commented that the stigma of marrying a person with epilepsy appears to be deep rooted in Chinese society, both in mainland China and in Taiwan. Thirty-one per cent (n=809) believed that people with epilepsy should not be employed in jobs as other persons are, and 7% (n=183) considered epilepsy to be a form of insanity. Thirty-four per cent (n=887) of the respondents did not know the cause of epilepsy, 28% (n=731) believed that epilepsy was a hereditary disease, 20% (n=522) believed that epilepsy was caused by brain disease or injury, 8% (n=209) believed that epilepsy was a mental or emotional disorder and 14% (n=365) believed that epilepsy was caused by birth defect. As for the clinical presentation of epilepsy, 13% (n=339) were not familiar with the nature of an epileptic attack, whereas 61% (n=1,592) identified convulsions and shaking movements and 52% (n=1,357) identified loss of consciousness as the typical manifestations of an epileptic seizure. Only 19% (n=496) recognised transient change of behaviour and 10% (n=261) recognised periods of amnesia as possible manifestations of an epileptic attack. Regarding treatment of epilepsy, 18% (n=47) did not know what to recommend if their friends or relatives had epilepsy. Sixty-three per cent (n=1,644) believed epilepsy should be treated by medical doctors and 15% (n=39) believed that epilepsy should be treated by herbal medicine doctors. Youth, higher education and upper levels of employment were correlated with answers that were more favourable concerning epilepsy in all survey questions except for the question regarding marriage, where the reverse was noted. Overall, the respondents' attitudes towards epilepsy in this Taiwan population were more negative than those obtained in the United States study, but more favourable than those detected in a similar survey conducted by Lai et al. (1990) in Henan Province in mainland China.

The study of a Chinese population by Lai et al. (1990) showed more negative attitudes towards epilepsy than in other countries. The reasons suggested for this discrepancy were less exposure to Western culture and a different socio-economic system. While the size of the sample was not specified, it was reported that 93% of those surveyed had heard or read about epilepsy, 77% knew someone with epilepsy and 72% had witnessed a seizure. Forty per cent did not know the cause of epilepsy, while 17% believed that epilepsy was a mental or emotional disorder. However, 57% said they would object to their child associating with someone with epilepsy, 87% would object to their child marrying a person with epilepsy, 53% thought their employment should be restricted and 16% regarded epilepsy as a form of insanity. Education was found to reduce prejudice but did not lessen the objections to marriage which may be linked to the finding that epilepsy was perceived as equating to insanity. The comparisons suggest that the exposure to Western culture and the socioeconomic system in Taiwan might have helped reduce the discrimination against epilepsy. The stigma of marrying persons with epilepsy appears to be deeply rooted in Chinese society, both in mainland China and in Taiwan. Regarding the treatment of epilepsy, fewer respondents from Taiwan (18%) than from China (39%) favoured Chinese herbal medicine and acupuncture as a treatment for epilepsy. This may also be related to the Taiwanese early exposure to multiple cultures in the past 400 years, as Taiwan was first discovered by Portuguese sailors in 1557, then ruled by Dutch (1661-1895), by Japanese (1895-1945) and later by the pro-west capitalist Nationalist Chinese (1945 to the present) (Su, 1986). As a result, the Taiwanese have had more exposure to Western medicine and are less influenced by Chinese orthodox medicine than are the Chinese of mainland China.

In a study of socialisation patterns among 15 university students with epilepsy in Canada, Andermann and Andermann (1992) reported that the students were selective about imparting knowledge about their seizures to fellow students, staff and employers, and most preferred not to volunteer information except to a close circle of friends. Half (53%) of the subjects felt that the discovery of their epilepsy had not interfered with their education in any way. If the diagnosis occurred in elementary school or early in high school, the teachers were usually made aware of the condition and were reported as understanding. However, elementary and high school classmates were not always as understanding, and this caused problems for several of the subjects. By the time they were attending college, most of these conflicts had been resolved and the subjects had developed a close circle of friends who knew about their epilepsy. However, all the subjects were aware of prejudices in society about epilepsy and believed that further education of the public was needed to improve the situation. They reported that young people with epilepsy are less well accepted by employers and co-workers in menial jobs, as found from their experience with summer employment. Thus, the authors concluded that the need for higher education is greater for people with epilepsy than for their non-epileptic siblings and peers.

Holdsworth and Whitmore (1974), in a survey of the information and attitudes held by head-teachers and class teachers in 60 mainstream schools that had children with epilepsy, found that in general they were sympathetic towards the children and anxious to treat the children as normally as possible. When asked if they were uneasy about, disliked or accepted having in their school a child who might have a seizure, only 3.3% (n=2) said they would prefer not to admit a child subject to major fits. The reason given by one was that he did not know what to do in the event of a major seizure and the other teacher said their school was over-crowded. A third head-teacher said that acceptance would depend upon the severity of the epilepsy. This question elicited a certain amount of anxiety among a few of the other 57 head-teachers, all of whom had at some time accepted a child subject to major fits. Two of them said they would have felt easier about admitting such a child had they known what to do in the event of a major seizure. Three others were less concerned about the possibility of seizures than about general management because of what they had been told by the parents. One mother had told the teacher that her son, who was subject to temporal lobe epilepsy, ".. had serious epilepsy, especially if he gets excited. He is to lead as normal a life as possible and so he does what he thinks he can." The boy's mother was also subject to epilepsy and a younger sister had died in status epilepticus during the survey year. The father of another boy had told the head-teacher that his son "was not well; he should not be frustrated and never punished." The doctor had told the third teacher that the girl should be "left to thrash around" when she had a fit. This teacher was uneasy about the possible consequences should a fit occur, for example, during a domestic science class. Two head-teachers revealed their anxiety and limited knowledge of epilepsy by explaining why they were less demanding of the child with epilepsy. One said he "adopted a greater degree of gentleness" in his approach, by which he meant that he would be less "blunt" than usual in asking for poor work to be re-done and tended "not to demand more of the child." The other teacher said that he did not ask the child to repeat poor work, nor did he give him homework, because he feared "such stress" might precipitate a seizure (although the boy did not have frequent fits and had never had one in school). Holdsworth and Whitmore (1974) felt that the tolerance of some head-teachers had misled them into accepting (perhaps even expecting) a lower level of work than they would have accepted had the child not been subject to epilepsy. Others who have studied children with epilepsy have voiced similar misgivings (Ounsted et al., 1966; Green and Hartlage, 1970).

Two young class-teachers were distinctly uneasy about having a child in their class who might have a major seizure because they had never seen a person in a convulsion. Another secondary-school head teacher said he was not sure how he and his school would stand up to the test of frequent disturbances caused by fits. Only five teachers said they thought the other children in the classes had been worried by the occurrence of a major fit. This was remarkable considering that 21% (n=18) of the children had had their first major seizure in school, which must have been a great surprise to both teachers and pupils. The children were said to be sympathetic, kind and tolerant when a child had a fit in school. One teacher said he thought that young children would not get used to fits occurring frequently, but many others told of how their pupils "got bored with it now" or "take it as a matter of course." One head-teacher who was unaware that a child had epilepsy until a seizure occurred in the school playground was calmly told by the children standing by that "she's having one of her turns, she often has them at home." An interesting example was a six-year old boy subject to major seizures whose classmates called him names and tended to shun him because of his aggressive behaviour. When one day he had a seizure in class and his difficulties were explained to the other children, the teacher reported that their attitudes became almost too tolerant!

Discussions with head-teachers and class-teachers revealed an over-simplified conception of epilepsy. Many retained lurid memories of grand mal seizures and hazy and mistaken ideas regarding management of a child with a convulsion. Not all were aware of petit mal epilepsy. Very few realised that it could be a serious educational disability, and if mentioned at all it was usually with little more interest than might have been shown about hay-fever. Although many teachers were aware of the need to exercise a degree of vigilance when children with epilepsy were in engaged in swimming, gymnastics, games and crafts requiring the use of cutting tools and hot appliances, the researchers felt that more awareness of potential danger would have been advisable in a few schools.

Bannon et al. (1992) undertook a survey of perceptions of childhood epilepsy among 142 mainstream teachers in North Staffordshire. Although this survey revealed more positive findings regarding teachers' perceptions than those found by Holdsworth and Whitmore (1974), only 5% (n=7) of the teachers reported that they felt 'very confident' when dealing with children who had epilepsy, 31% (n=44) felt 'quite confident' and 64% (n=90) replied that they 'did not feel confident.' Teachers who had previously witnessed a seizure had significantly higher levels of confidence. Similarly, confidence was higher in those who had a friend or relative who had epilepsy. Only 4% (n=5) of teachers felt that they knew enough about childhood epilepsy, 87% (n=120) considered their knowledge inadequate, and the remaining 9% (n=12) were not sure. Forty-six per cent of the teachers (n=66) stated that their confidence would be increased by further training and 44% (n=63) required more information in the form of booklets and leaflets. Despite this lack of confidence and specific training, the respondents demonstrated good general knowledge of epilepsy and adequate awareness of the difficulties encountered by schoolchildren with epilepsy. However, Bannon et al. (1992) believe that if optimal care is to be achieved for children with epilepsy, then teachers must feel confident with the condition. They feel that school health services have a clear role in ensuring that teachers have sufficient knowledge and adequate support.

The results of a transnational survey conducted in the Netherlands and the United Kingdom by de Boer et al. (1994) clearly illustrates how attitudes toward people with epilepsy are influenced by the degree of knowledge of the condition. Among a group of professionals (psychologists, occupational physicians, vocational therapists and social workers), 15% (n=11) of respondents believed in the existence of an 'epileptic personality'. After participants were educated about epilepsy, this figure declined to 6% (n=5).

An overview of the research on attitudes to epilepsy certainly indicates that adults and children with the disorder have to suffer some degree of stigmatisation and misunderstanding. However, the studies cited above show an improvement in public attitudes to epilepsy in a number of countries. Dinnage (1986) states that it would appear that the average person dealing with a child with epilepsy is nervous about fits, uncertain about what people with epilepsy are capable of accomplishing and ignorant about the spectrum of disability subsumed in the one word 'epilepsy'. She advises that education of public opinion should be directed towards showing how large a proportion of those suffering from epilepsy lead a normal and productive life.

3.4   EPILEPSY AND EMPLOYMENT

McLin and de Boer (1995) believe that the place of the worker often speaks volumes about society's views concerning a particular disability. They state that unemployment and under-employment are problems for people with epilepsy worldwide. According to Hall et al. (1997), those who do work tend to enter their profession or trade at a low level and tend to stay there. They are inclined to accept jobs without responsibility, and often deal with prejudice from employers by concealing their condition. Employers are frequently perceived as hostile and there is evidence of justification of this belief as they are often ill informed about epilepsy (Scrambler, 1993). A survey of members of the British Epilepsy Association showed that employment was the main area in which they experienced prejudice (Chappell, 1992). Few employers, including health authorities, have established policies on employing people with epilepsy, and even fewer follow guidelines (Floyd et al., 1993).

In their study of patient perceptions of their condition, Hayden et al. (1992) reported that 46% (n=238) of participants perceived employment as one of their major problems. However, the authors commented that employment is always a disputed issue, since whilst there is evidence of some discrimination, especially in difficult economic times, it is not surprising that employers are not over enthusiastic about employing staff with a medical problem. Furthermore, Hayden et al. (1992) believe that some people with epilepsy may have associated physical and personality problems and it could be these factors that, in fact, prevent gainful employment. In view of efforts to dispel the notion of the 'epileptic personality', this reference to the existence of 'personality problems' among people with epilepsy is quite surprising and could lead people to believe that all people with epilepsy have associated characteristics. Hayden et al. (1992) feel it is quite common for such persons to blame their epilepsy alone for their difficulties.

It is of interest that Hicks and Hicks (1991) reported that data from the U.S.A. shows an improvement in attitude towards the employment of persons with epilepsy over the past 30 years. However, in 1986 it was estimated that between 50,000 and 100,000 people in Britain were experiencing difficulties in finding or maintaining a job because of their epilepsy (Floyd, 1986). There are no similar figures for Ireland, but judging from anecdotal information Carroll (1992) believes that it is unlikely that they would differ radically. At a workshop held by Brainwave, the Irish Epilepsy Association, on Epilepsy Awareness Day in September 1998, the researcher noted that most of the young people in her group (n=30), stated that they can't get jobs when they mention they have epilepsy. They also commented that because they can't get employment they lose contact with friends.

Carroll (1992) conducted a follow-up review of 38 trainees who had completed social skill training programmes run by Brainwave, the Irish Epilepsy Association, and FAS, the Irish State training and employment authority, during the period 1986 to 1990. It was found that 61% (n=23) were unemployed, 16% (n=6) were in full-time employment, 3% (n=1) were in a part-time job and 21% (n=8) were in training. Fifty per cent (n=19) of those interviewed felt that they were being actively discriminated against because of their epilepsy. Carroll (1992) commented that it is not surprising, given these attitudes, that people with epilepsy do not wish to disclose information about their condition. According to McLellan (1987), people are usually willing and indeed relieved to disclose that they are sufferers, if they can be assured that they will be treated fairly.

For the young person with epilepsy in Ireland, especially when they continue to have seizures (no matter how occasional), employment prospects, are bleak (Carroll, 1992; Ross and Tookey, 1988; Andermann and Andermann, 1992). Ross and Tookey (1988) believe that only those with a good education will be in a favourable position to take up employment. Carroll (1992) concluded that the findings of her follow-up survey illustrated the need for a more comprehensive programme of training and development for young people with epilepsy in Ireland, many of whom are not being catered for under the existing rehabilitation programmes. Andermann and Andermann (1992) also stress that the need for higher education is greater for people with epilepsy compared with their non-epileptic siblings and peers. They believe that higher education increases self-esteem, improves chances of success in the working environment and should be encouraged whenever possible.

3.5   FACTORS INFLUENCING SOCIETY'S ATTITUDES

Although society's attitude to epilepsy is improving, and epilepsy may be more widely understood than formerly, much fear remains (Bagley, 1972). According to Gordon and Sillanpaa (1997), some of this fear is due to ignorance, but a certain amount is also due to a natural alarm when anyone suddenly suffers a loss of control. There is no doubt that epileptic seizures can be alarming, but society's views of epilepsy are to some extent shaped by a number of issues, in particular the type of seizure and indeed the person's own attitude to their condition.

3.5.1 Type of Epilepsy

According to Gordon and Sillanpaa (1997), the type of epilepsy and any associated disabilities may affect society's concepts of people who have epileptic seizures. For example, they explain that when seizures arise in the temporal lobes the person's behaviour may be awkward and difficult to control. This may be due to the attack itself, but more often the abnormal behaviour and the seizures are the result of damage to the temporal lobes. Frontal-lobe seizures can also cause bizarre manifestations as well as automatism, arrest of speech and spontaneous utterances (Brett and Neville, 1997). Prejudice may arise when behavioural problems or mental disabilities are seen in one individual with epilepsy and thought to apply to all people who have seizures. Gordon and Sillanpaa (1997) stress that such attitudes can only be corrected by more widespread knowledge of the clinical manifestations of epilepsy and the assertion that it is a common symptom of a wide variety of disorders, often with no recognisable cause. Sillanpaa (1992) advises that it is important to clarify that there are different types of seizures, with and without additional neurological deficits.

3.5.2 The Person's Own Attitude to Epilepsy

Gordon and Sillanpaa (1997) believe that an important factor affecting prejudice against those with epilepsy is the attitude of those who have the condition. They feel that if the individual can come to terms with the diagnosis of epilepsy and not let it affect their lives to too great an extent, the attitudes of others can be influenced. Conversely, if those with the condition become depressed, angry or unduly anxious, this will affect their own behaviour and the responses of others.

According to de Boer (1995), people with epilepsy can play an important role in educating the public about their condition, especially if they are reassuring, briefly describe their seizures and explain how it affects them and what can be done to help them. She stresses that it is of the utmost importance that people with epilepsy be taught how to talk about their condition in such a way that no matter which target group is involved, their audience should understand and therefore accept the condition and react appropriately when a seizure occurs. . De Boer (1995) compares education to a two-way street: people with epilepsy often demand understanding from the outside world, but they in turn should understand that witnessing a seizure may be a frightening experience for an uninformed bystander. When persons with epilepsy play their part well, they also play a vital and active role in improving mutual understanding between themselves and other members of society.

Gordon and Sillanpaa (1997) recommend that because attitudes are often established in childhood, information about epilepsy should be made available at an early age. In the case of young school children, the teacher is likely to play a key role. If a child has a seizure in class and the situation is dealt with in a matter-of-fact way without panic, the children will accept that there is nothing to be frightened of and understand that the affected child is liable to such attacks, and that they are in some way similar to fainting fits. Gordon and Sillanpaa (1997) stress that, for young children, the example set by the teacher is likely to have a significant effect. However, the teacher can only be expected to act in a calm and rational manner if in possession of sufficient knowledge to understand what is likely to happen and what should be done. They believe that it should be the responsibility of health workers, such as the school doctor or nurse, to impart the necessary information for each particular child with epilepsy.

3.5.3 Epilepsy in Literature
Literature often reflects society's attitudes, and superstition and prejudice against people with epilepsy often occurs in books and films (Paladin, 1995). Wolf (1998) believes that works of fiction may convey important information about images and public views of epilepsy. He notes that although some authors have done thorough research about epilepsy before writing, there are others whose knowledge of epilepsy stretches very little beyond some common prejudices which they uncritically repeat. Iliff (1998), in a review of a recent psychological thriller, 'Liar', writes that the ignorance and misunderstanding that still surrounds the condition in an apparently civilised society is highlighted in this film, with the police and health professionals wrongly interpreting the condition as sinister and dangerous. Throughout the film, epilepsy appears to be linked with mental illness, in particular psychosis. This link is reinforced by incidents such as the policemen consulting a psychiatrist, rather than a neurologist, in order to find out about the main character's condition. Iliff (1998) felt that the confusion the film engenders between epilepsy and psychosis is misleading, as people with no knowledge of epilepsy might assume the film was authoritative. The extreme and directed violence, along with the psychiatrist's opinion that "people with temporal lobe epilepsy make your skin crawl for a reason" might result in someone with no experience of the condition wrongly assuming that manipulative and violent characteristics are often associated with epilepsy. Films such as 'Liar' illustrate the attitudes that pertain, even today, towards epilepsy. Since feature films have a great impact on society, it is important that they portray epilepsy in a realistic, non-dramatic manner.

3.6 SUMMARY
This chapter examined public attitudes towards people with epilepsy and considered the contributory factors to these perceptions. According to McLin and de Boer (1995), sustained efforts by professional and voluntary organisations, as well as concerned individuals, have made major contributions to improving public perception about epilepsy and there is evidence that progress is being made. Nonetheless, they comment that those working in the field of epilepsy know that they are still far from fully demythologising and debunking long-held prejudices and

stigmas about the condition. The attitudes of society towards people with epilepsy, and vice versa, are extremely important, and the education of both parts is necessary. In society, there are various target groups such as parents, doctors, teachers and employers who require different information about epilepsy. Education for such target groups is organised by the national epilepsy associations in each country. In addition, the International Bureau for Epilepsy (IBE), the international umbrella organisation, which currently has over 50 national associations as members, is active in this field. Its goal, according to its constitution, is to improve the quality of life of all persons with epilepsy (de Boer, 1995). In Ireland, Brainwave, the Irish Epilepsy Association, provides information and advice to various target groups including parents, teachers and employers.

According to de Boer (1995), the attitudes of governments toward people with epilepsy and their care have been unduly influenced by financial considerations and ignorance of the precise nature of the condition. Pachlatko (1993) believes that over the centuries, economic factors, as well as negative attitudes towards epilepsy, have played an important role when dealing with governments. However, health care in general, as well as special epilepsy care, are becoming increasingly important issues for health ministers throughout the western world. For more than 100 years, limited organised epilepsy care has been offered in epilepsy centres in many European countries. However, institutionalisation, for both economical and psychosocial reasons, is no longer considered appropriate, and new models of care are being developed to correspond with modern views on epilepsy treatment. In the United Kingdom, Belgium and the Netherlands extended mobile outpatient clinics (EMOCs) have been created. The aims of such clinics are to offer specialised treatment and care to people with epilepsy to help them deal with daily life in society. De Boer (1995) considers EMOCs as clearly coinciding with developments in general health care and being in tune with ethical and economic considerations. She reports that the number of patient referrals to special centers for inpatient treatment has decreased in regions where such EMOCs operate and that they have been welcomed by national patient organisations. However, she argues that both economic and ethical considerations should complement one another in the development of epilepsy care services. Only then will epilepsy care services reach their primary goal: helping the person with epilepsy cope with daily life (de Boer, 1995).

Every year in Europe 240,000 babies who will later develop epilepsy are born (de Boer, 1995). It is for these infants that we should try to improve the living conditions of people with epilepsy by endeavoring to change attitudes and beliefs in society. Epileptic seizures do occur in society, and people with epilepsy are part of that society. Gordon and Sillanpaa (1997) stress that society's attitudes must be changed and to be effective this change must begin in schools. They believe that everyone involved with people with epilepsy should regard the eradication of prejudice as one of their responsibilities. A great deal can be achieved through efficient health education in informing the public about epilepsy. The use of materials such as films, programmes and packages about epilepsy for target groups, including teachers, pupils and employers, serve to heighten public awareness. Such initiatives are presently organised by Brainwave, the Irish Epilepsy Association. Similarly, training programmes for young people with epilepsy on presenting their condition to others will simultaneously serve to prepare them for dealing with prejudice and to educate the public about the condition. Such education and increased public awareness of the condition can help the child with epilepsy by dispelling long-held myths and attitudes.

CHAPTER FOUR

EPILEPSY AND FAMILY ADJUSTMENT

4.1   INTRODUCTION

Thompson and Upton (1992) comment on how epilepsy, unlike many other chronic disorders, is characterised by unpredictability and sudden onset of symptoms. Not only do seizures generally occur without warning, they can also take a variety of potentially embarrassing forms depending on the specific circumstances in which they occur. Clinical research by Thompson and Upton (1992) has shown that levels of stress may be elevated, not only in the person with epilepsy but also in family members, and that witnessing frequent seizures may be just as stressful as experiencing the seizure personally. However, the impact of epilepsy on the family, and the anxiety that it can engender for the parents or siblings of a child with epilepsy, have largely been ignored as a research topic. There is little evidence regarding the child and family's views (as opposed to those of professionals or researchers) on the effects of epilepsy on their lifestyle.

Aaronson (1988) reviewed the methodological pitfalls associated with the measurement of the concept of quality of life. He reported that a major problem with quality of life measurement is that it is often only defined in negative terms, that is, the absence of any physiological or psychological abnormality. Consequently, this approach is likely to underestimate the adverse changes for individuals with epilepsy who had previously been functioning within the superior or exceptional ability range prior to developing epilepsy. Aaronson (1988) also made two points of general importance: quality of life measurement is multidimensional, and perspectives on quality of life vary with the individual. Quality of life assessment will also vary according to the perspective of the observer, for instance the professional such as the doctor or social worker, the parents or the child.

Duncan (1990) also emphasised the multidimensional nature of quality of life assessment for people with epilepsy. He proposed four dimensions: neurological, psychological, social and occupational/educational. The neurological dimension involves the frequency and severity of seizures, any neurological deficit and the adverse effects from anticonvulsant medication. The psychological dimension assesses affective state, cognition and memory, while the social and educational/occupational dimensions concentrate on social relationships and progress at school or work, respectively.

Hoare and Russell (1995) describe an attempt to modify an existing questionnaire (Hoare, 1986, 1993) in order to provide a more comprehensive assessment of the impact of epilepsy on the quality of life of the child and family. The questionnaire assesses four aspects of the child and family's lifestyle: epilepsy and its treatment, impact on the child, impact on the parent and impact on the family. The authors concluded that results of the pilot validation study provided preliminary evidence to support the usefulness of the questionnaire. It is intended that further research will be undertaken to assess the usefulness of the questionnaire on a larger and more representative group of children with epilepsy.

This chapter reviews the findings of studies reporting on the adjustment of parents and siblings of children diagnosed with epilepsy. It examines the impact of the diagnosis on the parents, and the reactions it may evoke. The effect of the seizures on the family's social life, and restrictions which parents sometimes impose on the child with epilepsy are also documented. A review of both school-related and medical concerns which may be experienced by parents is included. The effects on other family members and parents' concerns regarding the future are also explored.

4.2   REACTIONS EVOKED BY THE DIAGNOSIS

It is a very emotional time when parents find out their child has epilepsy, whether it is at birth or during childhood. The impact of having a child with epilepsy may be significant medically, socially and psychologically. Family equilibrium may be affected, as most parents are overcome by feelings of grief, as well as experiencing fears and doubts about the future.

Although seizures occur before the diagnosis, these are usually regarded as 'episodes'; something is wrong, but no one is sure what it is (McGovern 1982). The reactions of the family to the diagnosis of epilepsy may produce feelings which are similar to those experienced in bereavement. Emotions of denial, panic, anger and sadness may all be felt in turn. The family responses may be considered under the following headings (Pond, 1979):
1.   Attitude to aetiology and hereditary factors
2.   Attitudes of parents to their sick child
3.   Attitudes of parents to treatment
4.   Attitudes of parents to doctors and other members of the medical team
5.   Attitudes of parents to each other and to the siblings, if any

The following are some of the most commonly experienced reactions of parents to the diagnosis of epilepsy.

Fear
Wallace (1994) notes that the initial seizure and subsequent attacks can often cause great fear, though later reactions may vary from total denial to suffocating over-protection. McGovern (1982) comments on how the effect of the diagnosis on the parents is most likely to be one of fear for the child and his future, and a feeling of inadequacy to cope with the diagnosis. Parents may also experience a vague and hesitantly expressed fear of an association between epilepsy and some degree of inevitable 'mental abnormality or retardation' (Ward and Bower, 1978). If the child is very young, or if the seizures are diagnosed as part of a more permanently disabling condition, a sense of bereavement may also be experienced (McGovern, 1982).
Pond (1981) and Hall et al. (1997) note that parents may fear that some failure of care on their part has precipitated the epilepsy. This could include fears about neglect during pregnancy, poor relationships with the child in infancy, accidents involving a head injury, infections of the brain, or emotional stress in the home.

Guilt
Many parents experience an unjustified sense of guilt, and torment themselves with self-questioning about the cause of their child's epilepsy (Green, 1985; McGovern, 1982). They wonder about hereditary factors, particularly if they themselves had convulsions in early childhood: a fact they may not have been aware of until grandparents, or other relations were asked about family history. McGovern (1982) considers that another equally destructive question is "Which side of the family did it come from?" Pond (1981) comments that if the cause is not known, the doctor may use the word 'idiopathic'. Parents are therefore left to speculate on whether they themselves may inadvertently have caused it, perhaps through psychological trauma to the child arising from their own inter-personal difficulties.

According to McGovern (1982) many fathers look on epilepsy in their child as a slur on their virility, particularly if the child is a son. There is often unspoken guilt in one or other of the parents, and this can threaten the relationship between husband and wife and ultimately, the structure of family life. Wallace (1994) advises genetic counselling for parents, notably those who have a history of epilepsy, since many affected mothers in particular, are likely to feel guilty and may be blamed by their partners for the child's epilepsy.

Denial
Pond (1981) describes how the initial diagnosis may be disturbing, as the word 'epilepsy' often conjures up the idea of a hereditary degenerative stigma. There may be denial, sometimes in collusion with the doctor, if parents are told that "It's just a convulsion." Often, as a continuation of early denial, the child will be expected to be 'normal' in every way. Pond (1981) comments that this can be beneficial in terms of encouraging self-reliance in children, and in encouraging responsibility for managing their own treatment. However, Pond (1981) warns that parental denial of the condition can be disastrous if the child's attainment in school is affected while he or she is nevertheless expected to maintain the same standard as their peers.

Overprotection
Overprotection is a common response to the diagnosis of epilepsy. The child may be so watched-over as to feel 'smothered', not mothered (Pond, 1981). Children can be over-indulged,

sometimes to the detriment of other family members. Over-protection and parental anxiety may lead to discipline problems, because parents may hesitate to use disciplinary measures, for fear that reprimands may provoke seizures (Wallace, 1994). This may also be a cause for marital disharmony, and the child may be handled inconsistently.

At times, the diagnosis may even be kept from the child. Pond (1981) refers to an intelligent man in his 30s whose ageing middle-class parents still looked after his drugs telling him he was a lifelong sufferer of migraine, not epilepsy! Extreme reactions always imply intense anxiety on the part of the parents.

Andermann and Andermann (1992), in a study of 15 students attending university in Montreal, Quebec found that, according to the subjects' point of view, the impact of the diagnosis of epilepsy on the parents consisted mainly of initial overprotection, followed by acceptance and support. In one case, however, a mother was said to feel guilty because she herself had epilepsy, making acceptance more difficult. The only exceptions were found in some southern European and Asian families, where culturally-determined secretive behaviour made life after the diagnosis much more difficult for the parents. They worried that news of their child's condition would spread through the ethnic community and possibly interfere with their child's chances for a good marriage. Siblings were said to respond with much less emotion. The reactions of all the children to their diagnoses were similar, consisting of a period of initial anger, depression and fear, which was then replaced by acceptance, achieved through an improved understanding of their condition and better medical control.

Rejection
Instead of denial and over-protection, McGovern (1982) comments that the immediate reaction could sometimes be that of rejection, in various forms. This could involve either temporary or permanent rejection of the child, acceptance of the child as 'second best', or acceptance of him as 'delicate' and in need of compensatory and special care. According to Pond (1981), it can sometimes be rejection of the disease itself, but more often it is of the unfortunate sufferer who may in some way be excluded by the family. This may include placement in a special school, or the opinion that the child is ineducable.

Relief
Occasionally the period of investigation causes such anxiety that the diagnosis of epilepsy may actually be received with relief because it explains a puzzling behavioural disturbance (McGovern, 1982; Green, 1985). Many parents fear that their child has a brain tumour and are relieved to learn that it is epilepsy.

4.3   THE IMPACT OF SEIZURES ON PARENTS
Ward and Bower (1978), in a study of the impact on parents of having a child with epilepsy, found that of the many fears aroused by a child's epilepsy, those engendered by the actual seizure is the most dominant. This fear is not confined to children who have major seizures, as the fear may extend to all types of seizures. Most parents experience a degree of fear and horror which may only diminish with increased confidence and familiarity. Ward and Bower (1978) identified the following features which parents find most frightening:

Death
Understandably, many parents think their child is dead on the first occasion that they witness a seizure (Clare et al., 1978; Green, 1985: Ward and Bower, 1978). Thompson and Upton (1992) found that a past record of status epilepticus was also associated with high levels of both anxiety and depression among the primary carers, the mother being the primary carer for 80% (n=35) of the families. The occurrence of such episodes would seem to reinforce a family's fear of death, a fear that has been reported to be high both in persons with epilepsy and in mothers of children with epilepsy (Hoare, 1986).

Breathing
Ward and Bower (1978) comment that although the diagnosis of epilepsy may allay the fear of death, this fear often persists because of the child's breathing difficulties during an attack. In their

study they reported that several parents expressed a fear of choking as a result of the supposed risk of swallowing the tongue, or apprehension concerning vomiting or a gurgling noise in the throat. Several fathers and one mother had their hands bitten when attempting to secure an airway by forcing the teeth apart. Many parents used the phrases "stops breathing" and "goes blue", and described the agony of suspense as they watched for the return of normal breathing and colour.

Loss of Consciousness
Fears related to loss of consciousness were also very prevalent among the parents in Ward and Bower's study (1978). This was also related to the fear of death during a seizure, but commonly it was expressed in terms of loss of contact with the child. The fear was not confined to the more severe seizures, because for some parents even a brief "switching off" provoked it. The parents of a thirteen year old girl whose minor seizures initially took the form of verbal amnesia and "talking nonsense," but later included "blanking-out" found the latter extremely frightening.

Other Fears
Other less dramatic features, which Ward and Bower (1978) found to provoke horror or distress among parents included:
Noise: Many parents reported lying awake awaiting "the noise" or initial cry that signaled the onset of an attack.
Salivation: 'Frothing' or 'foaming at the mouth' seemed to be especially horrifying, and to the lay mind was one of the features particularly associated with epilepsy. Parents who had seen this in their child usually mentioned it with revulsion, as something especially difficult to tolerate, and also as something which had indicated that the first episode was "some kind of fit". Conversely, others emphasised that salivation had not occurred, and therefore were 'reassured' that the episode could not have been a real fit or "real epilepsy."
Twisting and jerking: These features are also generally thought to be associated with epilepsy, and for some parents had provided the first indication of the nature of the episode. To some parents these features were frightening because they were suggestive of epilepsy, and in others they provoked particular fears and some revulsion.
Eye-movements and staring: Eye-rolling and fixation engendered similar fears. These may be related to the parental fear of unconsciousness as suggested by such phrases as "glassy-eyed", "looking through you" and "staring but not seeing." Sometimes there was a fear of disfigurement.
Incontinence: This was not regarded as a primary focus of anxiety or revulsion, probably because very few children are habitually incontinent during a seizure. However, parents are more likely to be anxious about it occurring in school.
Aura: Some children may experience fear either during an aura or minor seizure, and this can be very distressing to the parents.

Fear Of How To Cope
Apart from the fears related to specific features of the seizures, Ward and Bower (1978) commented there was also a frequently expressed fear of "how to cope" with a condition which they knew nothing about. Concerns included management of medication and procedures to be followed during and after a seizure. Understandably, this fear was most common among parents of newly diagnosed children and those who had not yet witnessed their child having a seizure (the seizures having occurred, for example, at school or while they were with relatives or friends).

Use of Specific Terminology
Ward and Bower (1978) noted that the terminology used by parents often gave an insight into their level of understanding and acceptance of the diagnosis. Parents tended to select terms and to make their own distinctions; for instance, for some a "convulsion" was not a "fit" and was therefore less frightening. For others the reverse applied, a "convulsion" being far worse than a "fit". Similarly, some said that "fits" were "not epileptic" or "not really epileptic"; others talked of "epilepsy", yet the episode was "not a proper fit". Sometimes such distinctions were reasonable, bearing in mind the strong correlation of epilepsy with 'grand mal' in the lay mind and the lack of knowledge about minor or absence seizures. The word 'epilepsy' had not always been used in medical explanations, so therefore, failure of parents to use it did not necessarily indicate rejection.

Ward and Bower (1978) noted that control of seizures appears to be the key factor in satisfactory management of children with epilepsy. Once the seizures are controlled, other fears can be coped with and adjustment made by the parents and the children themselves. Ward and Bower (1978) concluded that identification of vulnerable families needs much more time and care, and would probably be best achieved by a team approach based in special clinics for epilepsy. Such identification should be part of the initial referral and diagnosis procedure and should provide parents with the opportunity to express their emotions and concerns.

4.4   THE IMPACT OF EPILEPSY ON FAMILY LIFE

According to McGovern (1982), fear that a seizure may occur and embarrassment about public reactions can severely limit a family's social activities. Early onset intractable epilepsy accompanied by additional disabilities has a widespread effect on the child's and family's quality of life and overall adjustment Hoare (1993).

Hoare (1993), investigating the quality of life among 108 school children with chronic epilepsy in Edinburgh, found that epilepsy clearly had a very significant impact on the family. This was reflected by parental concerns expressed in several ways: the management of seizures, including the adverse side effects from anti-convulsants; the deleterious effects on the child's adjustment and development; and the restrictions on family life and activities. While the children in this study were not drawn from a total population of children with epilepsy, they were representative of children with the more severe and/or long-standing forms of epilepsy in the region.

Ferrari et al. (1983) studied 45 children aged six to 12 years, and their families, to examine the effects the child's illness had on family functioning. The children were divided into three groups of 15: children with epilepsy, children with diabetes and children without chronic illness. Tests of adjustment and self-concept were administered at home to all the children and family members. The children with epilepsy were reported by parents to differ from the other two groups in a number of ways: they were more inclined to complain of rejection, to act in an immature manner, to have periods of emotional stress and to be aggressive towards their parents. Regarding the question of family cohesion, the families of children with epilepsy reported themselves to be significantly less close than families in the two other groups. The children with epilepsy showed a lower self-concept than the other two groups of children. Ferrari et al. (1983) concluded that it appears that there is a particular set of characteristics associated with epilepsy that distinguishes it from other chronic illness.

McGovern (1982) describes how the effect of the seizure (not only the period of the actual physical 'absence' or partial seizure but the anticipation of it) can be of major concern for the family. During the day there is the constant worry about where the child is, and what risks might arise from that situation. Even when the child is in school, some parents will always be expecting a telephone call informing them that their child has had a seizure, and perhaps requesting them to collect him/her. Similar tension may arise if the parents become unduly anxious about the child during the night to the extent that they take it in turns to sleep with the child in case she/he has a seizure. Many parents feel they are 'on call' 24 hours a day, without a break. Not surprisingly, these tensions can greatly affect the relationship between the couple. The condition can be a focus for conflict, with higher rates of separation and divorce (Betts, 1993). The National Child Development Study (NCDS) in Britain found that, as a group, one-parent families of children with epilepsy were over-represented, and that divorce and death of one parent, particularly fathers, was more common than expected (Ross et al. 1980).

McGovern (1982) warns that there is the risk that the family of a child with epilepsy will close in on itself and that the child with epilepsy will become the pivot around which family life revolves. She adds that the practice of closing ranks gives rise to a multitude of problems because the child who is overprotected may find it very difficult to relate to others and will live with a sense of shame or a consciousness of 'being different'. For the parents, the act of closing ranks can cut them off from adult company and narrow their horizons and opportunities, which in turn will adversely affect the atmosphere in the home. Wallace (1994) comments that many parents are reluctant to spend an evening out socially together because of difficulties with delegating care to relatives or minders. If the child has difficult seizures, people are generally reluctant to offer to look after them. However, McGovern (1982) advises that if friends can see how the family copes with a seizure they will be more likely to be prepared to take over from time to time. The alternative to this is to leave the older children in charge. Here McGovern (1982) also warns that this is a sensitive area of family management and one that needs special consideration so that siblings do not feel resentful about it.

Many parents of children with epilepsy feel a great deal of dissatisfaction about their lack of a social life. Thompson and Upton (1992) found that 68% (n=30) of primary carers were dissatisfied with aspects of their social life. Primary carers were defined as the people responsible for taking on the major task of supporting the person with epilepsy; for 80% (n=35) of the families in their study, the mother was considered the primary carer. All of the carers reported that they experienced most problems in the area of limited social activities and intimate relationships. Questions regarding the lifestyle of the carer suggested little respite from the caring role, and a wish for some respite from that role was expressed. Fifty-nine per cent (n=26) of the primary carers reported engaging in social and leisure activities less than once a month, while 71% (n=31) of them had not spent a night away from the person with epilepsy in the previous year. Seventy-three per cent (n=32) of primary carers also reported that they had not had a holiday without the individual with epilepsy in the last five years. The majority of primary carers rated the level of support they received as limited. This lack of practical assistance from social and other State services, and a lack of emotional support from a partner were seen to be significantly associated with poor emotional adjustment and high levels of anxiety and depression among the primary carers. Analysis of the relationship between the nature of the epilepsy and the emotional state of the primary carers factors yielded three significant results: (1) raised levels of anxiety were associated with severity of tonic and atonic seizures and frequency of episodes of status epilepticus; (2) elevated levels of depression were associated with increased frequency of status epilepticus and (3) no other seizure or medication variables examined were significantly associated with the psychological state of the primary carer. Analysis of the perceived level of support received from services showed that the lower the reported practical support, the higher the reported levels of depression. Similarly, there was a significant relationship between emotional support received from the spouse and level of depression in the primary carer.

4.5 RESTRICTIONS IMPOSED BY PARENTS AND OTHER PROFESSIONALS

Over-protection of the child with epilepsy frequently involves restrictions which limit the child's ability to perform daily activities in the manner, or within the range, considered appropriate. According to Pond (1981), parents may impose restrictions to reduce the risk of seizure-related injuries because of their fear of seizures occurring in potentially dangerous situations. He comments that many parents worry when their child is five minutes late from school that he or she is under a bus. Many parents insist that the bedroom door is left open so that nocturnal fits can be heard and attended to, or the child can be watched unobtrusively and regularly in case he is suffocating. The child's response to these restrictions is variable. Some rebel, especially in adolescence, and tantrums and violence may result. Others comply more or less reluctantly, and this may contribute to the passivity or withdrawal which characterises some chronic epilepsy (Pond, 1981).

Restrictions can sometimes adversely influence the development of children with epilepsy and result in underachievement in school and delay in personal development (Thompson and Oxley, 1993). According to Mitchell et al. (1994), sociocultural factors are the most important cause of anxiety and negative attitudes in the parents of children with epilepsy. Some parents may not wish their children to know that they have epileptic seizures because they dread the stigma and prejudice attached to the diagnosis. This attitude is understandable but Gordon and Sillanpaa (1997) advise that to keep the diagnosis from teachers and other carers may be unwise, particularly if the child is taking anti-epileptic drugs.

Long and Moore (1979), in a study of parental expectations for their child with epilepsy, reported that there was a significant difference between parents' expectations for the child with epilepsy and his or her siblings. Parents saw themselves as more dominant and strict when dealing with the child with epilepsy. The majority thought that he or she should be supervised at all times: swimming, cycling, team games and climbing were prohibited in 28, 21, 16 and 11 per cent of cases respectively. More of the children with epilepsy than of the controls were described as socially isolated. Self-esteem scores were lower for the children with epilepsy. Parents' and teachers' ratings of psychiatric disturbance indicated that they found the children with epilepsy to be more disturbed than their siblings. The authors concluded that parents can influence their children for the worse by their expectations, and that more advice and information from medical professionals about appropriate restrictions are needed.

Pond (1981) describes how both doctors and teachers may also unwittingly reinforce parents' anxiety over the dangers of physical exercise, especially in relation to swimming and gym. Carpay et al. (1997) found that the neurologists had advised imposing restrictions on about two-thirds (66%) of the 122 children in their study. This advice was shown to have a significant influence on the parents, because parent-reported disability among the children due to restrictions was reported in 83% (n=101) of the children. 'Disability' was defined by the authors as any restriction or lack of ability to perform an activity in the manner or within the range considered normal for a human being. The authors recommended that counselling about restrictions be repeated at regular intervals for the parents of any child with epilepsy, because during the course of treatment, the child's symptoms and type of epilepsy may change.

Holdsworth and Whitmore (1974), in their study of children with epilepsy attending mainstream schools, reported that head-teachers had imposed restrictions on 31% (n=26) of children. Restrictions had more often been imposed on children subject to major attacks (34%) than on those with 'petit-mal' (20%), but they did not seem to be related to frequency of seizures. Half the children with frequent seizures, including two with weekly seizures, were not under any restriction. Of the 26 children subject to restrictions, 69% (n=18) were not allowed to swim; 15% (n=4) were excluded from certain activities in physical education, whereas 12% (n=3) others were excluded from all forms of physical education; 19% (n=5) children were restricted in other ways: 8% (n=2) were not allowed to cycle to school and 8% (n=2) were not permitted by their head-teachers to undertake assignments outside school. Of these two, one was not allowed to take part in cross-country running because of the school's earlier experience with another boy who had a seizure during a run. Two secondary-school pupils had been excluded from school expeditions involving over-night stays. It was noted that all senior pupils took an active part in crafts, home economics, wood and metal–work classes.

Tattenborn and Kramer (1992) advise that restrictions imposed by teachers should be minimal. Such restrictions, compounded by teasing by other pupils, can have a profound effect on the child's feelings of self-esteem and consequently on their behaviour (Besag, 1995). In general, bullying and teasing of children with epilepsy are particularly evident in secondary schools (Wilde and Haslam, 1996). This may occur because it is so important during adolescence not to appear different in any way and peers are likely to be less tolerant.

According to Ward and Bower, (1978) some parents may avoid making any restrictions, even where these may be desirable because of the nature and frequency of the child's seizure. They comment that this is probably the result of a strong drive to prove their child's 'normality'.

Green (1985) argues that restrictions imposed on children with epilepsy should vary according to intellectual capacity, behaviour and type and frequency of seizure, and should relate to a child's individual risk profile. A child will be more at risk of getting injured due to a seizure when they are frequent, severe or unpredictable. However, in a comparative study of quality of life of childhood epilepsy and asthma, Austin et al. (1994) found that a score reflecting participation in social activities did not correlate with seizure frequency. Parents may impose restrictions simply because their child has a disorder, regardless of the specific risks associated with the medical condition. Austin et al. (1994) also found that social activity scores did not differ significantly between children with epilepsy and asthma.

It has been suggested that the age of the child (Freeman, 1987) and the presence of other impairments (Sillanpaa, 1992; Hauser, 1994) may often influence the necessity of restrictions. Despite the lack of specific risk profiles, most authors (O'Donohue, 1983; Green, 1985; Sonnen, 1988; Engel, 1989; Aicardi, 1994) agree about the need for global guidelines concerning restrictions in childhood epilepsy. Activities for which restrictions are often advised are bathing, swimming, climbing and cycling. According to Aicardi (1994), everyday life at home should not be restricted except for children with especially dangerous types of seizures. Participation in sports and physical exercise is generally not discouraged. Sonnen (1988) advises that parents, with the advice of their child's doctor, must set the standard of acceptable risk and make their own judgements.

According to Carpay et al. (1997), the importance of minimising restrictions on the child's daily activities should be emphasised, as many parents may be reluctant to encourage independence in the child for fear of the consequences. They stress that doctors, particularly paediatricians, have an important role to play in minimising restrictions and in encouraging the parents to allow appropriate independence to develop. Parents are likely to benefit from specific practical advice, which should be monitored, adjusted and given on set occasions so that ambiguities and uncertainties can be clarified. This approach is likely to enhance parents' confidence in their upbringing of their child and reduce the burden for both the child and the family.

4.6   SCHOOL-RELATED CONCERNS

Hoare (1984b) reports that schooling is often a particular source of concern for children with epilepsy. Parents worry whether the epilepsy is adversely affecting the child's work and behaviour at school, and fearfully watch for signs of reduced performance. Conversely, some parents may deny intellectual retardation despite firm evidence of learning difficulties (Ward and Bower, 1978).

Bannon et al. (1992) comment that although epilepsy is a common disorder, it still retains a social stigma that may result in parental reluctance to share information with teaching staff. Parents may wish to keep their child's epilepsy a secret, and this poses a potential danger to the child and problems for school staff if they have not been told about and prepared for seizures which may occur (Ross and Tookey, 1988). According to Pond (1981), parents are often anxious about rejection arising from the attitudes of others. These apprehensions range from fear of teasing by other children to fear of rejection by the school.

Holdsworth and Whitmore (1974b), in a study of 85 children attending 60 mainstream schools in England, reported that the head teachers had been informed about the epilepsy of 62% (n=53) of the children, but were initially unaware of it in a further 35% (n=30) of the group. Reliable information regarding two children was not made available. The head teachers first became aware that 21% (n=18) of the children had epilepsy when they had seizures in school; for two children this was the first manifestation of their epilepsy. It was quite by chance that another five children were revealed to have epilepsy. In one case, the head teacher had called the police in to deal with a child reported to be taking drugs in the toilet; it was then discovered that he had been taking his anti-epileptic medication. Seven additional children were brought to the notice of the head teachers as a result of Holdsworth and Whitmore's survey.

In the case of 53 children whose teachers had been informed of their epilepsy, there were 64% (n=34) whose parents, school doctors or previous head teachers had told the present teachers of the type of seizure to expect. This information was not available for the remaining 36% (n=19) children, or for the 9% (n=5) whose epilepsy had come to light by chance when the survey began. Thus of the 58 children whose head teachers knew of their epilepsy before the sudden onset of a seizure, there were 41% (n=24) of teachers who were ignorant as to the type of seizure likely to occur.

In 13% (n=8) of the 60 schools, the head teacher did not know what to do if a child had a seizure. In the other 87% (n=52) of schools, the head teacher (but not the class teacher) knew what to do if a child had a major seizure. They usually knew what to do from previous experience, or from general knowledge or first-aid training. In some cases they only knew from what the parents had told them, though occasionally the parents were even more uninformed! Somewhat unorthodox parental tips on management of seizures included: "Put his feet in warm water and loosen his clothing"; "He rolls on the floor – put a spoon in his mouth and leave him"; "Smack her if she has a fit" and "Pour cold water over him".

Holdsworth and Whitmore (1974b) were disturbed to discover that communication between teachers and school doctors about pupils with epilepsy was the exception rather than the rule. The

School Health Service had known of 71% (n=60) of the children. In 8% (n=5) of cases, these had only come to the notice of the services when the children were having their school-leaving medical examination. However, the School Health Service had informed the head teachers of only 40% (n=22) of these 55 children. They were aware of three of the five children whom the teachers had discovered by chance, and all seven children who were revealed as a result of the survey.

Although the survey conducted by Bannon et al. (1992) revealed more positive findings regarding communication between parents and teachers, the authors were disappointed that this aspect of the care of children with epilepsy had not improved greatly since the study by Holdsworth and Whitmore (1974b). Of the 142 mainstream teachers surveyed in North Staffordshire, it was found that of the 81 teachers who to their knowledge had taught a child with epilepsy, 49% (n=40) were first made aware of it by prior discussion with parents. However, 30% (n=24) first learned of the child's epilepsy when the child had a seizure in school, and 14% (n=11) of teachers had discussion with either the school nurse or doctor. In general, teachers welcomed the notion of prior discussion with parents and they considered frequency of fits, medication, warning signs of imminent fits and parent contact details to be essential. Bannon et al. (1992) suggested that this lack of communication could be improved if hospital paediatricians had a close liaison with colleagues in the School Health Service. School nurses, in particular, are in a good position to ensure that adequate communication exists between parents, school and hospital services. The 'parent-held' child health record has already been shown to improve communication between parents and other parties and could be of great benefit in the area of epilepsy (MacFarlane, 1992).

Hanai (1996), in a study of the quality of life in school children with epilepsy in Japan, surveyed families and teachers of 344 elementary and junior high school children with epilepsy. Of these children, 73% (n=252) attended ordinary classes, whereas 27% (n=92) received education for disturbed children in special classes or schools. The major concerns of families regarding their children were seizures and the future of their child. Higher rates of concern regarding forgetting to take medicine and 'school records' were noted among the children in Group A (those attending ordinary classes). (It was not explained what "school records" meant, but it possibly meant academic progress). Higher rates of concern for the future, health conditions other than seizures and relationships with brothers and sisters were noted in Group B (special) than in Group A (mainstream). Regarding the character and behaviour characteristics of children with epilepsy, many parents answered: "I do not think there are such characteristics or behaviors", but 9% (n=163) of teachers and 29% (n=100) of families said there were. The major comments from teachers regarding children with epilepsy included "being restless," "taking frequent naps," and "being fickle", whereas families reported characteristics such as "being restless," "being persistent," "being short-tempered" and "being exact." Some of these items appeared to be associated with seizure intractability, associated handicaps, seizure frequency or side effects of anti-epileptic drugs (AEDs). In Group A (mainstream), 26% (n=66) of families explained the epilepsy to the children in detail, 23% (N=58) explained a little and 31% (n=78) explained only that seizures occurred. In Group B (special), 11% (n=10) explained in detail, 17% (n=16) explained a little, but 63% (n=58) indicated that they hadn't explained epilepsy, saying that the children couldn't understand even if they did explain. The most common concerns regarding school for families of children with epilepsy were to do with inability to keep up, difficulty in making friends and being easily tormented. In Group B (special), seizures occurring at school and children frequently requiring a nap were major concerns of parents. Schools were informed of the name of the child's condition by 91% (n=84) of families in Group B (special) but by only 48% (n=121) of families in Group A (mainstream). This was probably due to the fact that the severity of epilepsy and related conditions was clearly higher in Group B. Reasons for families not informing schools about their child's condition included: fear of prejudices and discrimination, concern about restraints being placed on their child's participation in physical education and in school events, privacy being infringed, confidentiality being insufficient and the child's future being affected. Concerning participation in physical education and school events, 55% (n=994) of teachers and 60% (n=206) of families responded that children should participate in all activities under particular conditions relating to the individual child if seizures could be controlled. More families than teachers agreed that, regardless of whether seizures are controlled, children should participate in all activities with proper regard being paid to individual considerations, and this response was more frequent among teachers in schools for handicapped children and families among Group B (special). However, a large number of teachers responded that even if seizures can be controlled, prohibition is necessary for some sports such as swimming. From the results of the survey, teachers in schools for handicapped children appeared to have more knowledge of epilepsy and seizures than teachers in mainstream schools. This was probably because they had more contact with children with epilepsy and had received training in that area. Hanai (1996) stressed the importance of the role of the school teacher in the management and education of the child with epilepsy, and advised that it might be necessary to strengthen education on epilepsy and behavioural disturbances in the training curriculum for teachers and to add such topics to postgraduate training.

From the research evidence, it would appear that schools, and particularly teachers, have an important role to play in facilitating the successful adjustment of the child with epilepsy and his parents to the condition and to school. Schools can reduce parents' anxieties and encourage independence and self-esteem if they are knowledgeable about epilepsy and its treatment. This necessitates education of the teaching and support staff in the individual needs of each child with epilepsy. The difficulties which can arise may be minimised by school awareness, development of strategies for coping with seizures, the acknowledgement that there may be special educational needs and planning for employment. Total avoidance of subject-areas such as computers on the basis of epilepsy which is not proven to be photosensitive can unnecessarily restrict the curriculum (Wallace, 1994).

Paediatricians and school medical doctors should ensure that teachers are informed in these matters, so that appropriate attitudes and patterns of care for the child with epilepsy are adopted. Following the initial diagnosis, both the medical professionals and the health board should contact the child's teacher with specific details regarding the child's condition. Close liaison between doctors and schools is essential if the child with epilepsy is to make satisfactory progress at school. Ross and Tookey (1988) have stressed that doctors must encourage parents to inform their child's school about their condition and that doctors should contact the school by means of letter, telephone call and even a visit. Doctors should explain to parents that there may be no simple answers to behavioural and cognitive problems, and that not only the possible effects of the epilepsy itself, but also the complex interactions of anticonvulsant therapy, must be considered if there are educational and behavioural difficulties.

4.7 THE EFFECT OF EPILEPSY ON OTHER FAMILY MEMBERS

Epilepsy in a child has an inevitable impact on family dynamics. McGovern (1982) cautions that the formal diagnosis using the actual word "epilepsy" might affect other family members in various ways. She adds that grandparents may possibly be affected very deeply if they hold the 'old fashioned view' of the condition being something to be ashamed of and wish to hush it up and pretend it hasn't happened. However, it is often the grandparents who witness seizures prior to the diagnosis and who are the first people to suspect the nature of the condition because they have had previous experience of epilepsy. Ward and Bower (1978) reported that 26% (n=21) of the parents of children with epilepsy whom they interviewed thought that there had been excessive reactions by relatives, some being frightened of the seizures and of having to cope with them.

It is becoming more widely recognised that the siblings of the child with epilepsy may also be at risk because of distortions in the family dynamics (Rutter et al. 1971; Hoare, 1984a; Hoare, 1984b; McGovern, 1982; Ferrarri et al. 1983; Hoare and Kerley, 1991). This is not only because the child with epilepsy tends to dominate the family scene, but also because the innermost feelings of the brothers or sisters often remain unspoken. McGovern (1982) emphasises that life both at home and at school can be difficult for the siblings of children with epilepsy. At school they may have to cope with their brother or sister during a seizure, or live with the attitudes of others. At home, parents may be worried and anxious, and because the children don't want to increase their burden, they conform. They may have a legitimate need to discuss their own worries, ambitions, school problems, and arguments with friends with their parents, but they decide not to add further to their anxieties. They cope by bottling up their problems, which may sometimes erupt in bursts of anti-social behaviour, moods, or classic cries for help in the form of petty stealing or bed-wetting (McGovern, 1982). She also warns that they may become frightened, not only of the seizures, but of their own feelings. Family holidays ruined, parties and visits cut short or outings cancelled are difficult for siblings to understand and accept, particularly if everyone else appears to take the disruptions for granted. Resentment may gradually build up and, because it is difficult for children to be objective, it may not always be against the epilepsy but against the child with epilepsy. They may harbour feelings of anger and frustration that can cause them to react negatively to their brother or sister. Feelings of guilt will follow, and these can be very damaging if not discussed. Parents often assume that everyone in the family can cope and children may feel guilty if they can't. According to McGovern (1982), epilepsy in the family can alter the roles played by various members, and so change relationships. If the mother's attention is exclusively on the child with epilepsy, the older children may become responsible for the younger ones. Alternatively, the child with epilepsy may become the special responsibility of his brother or sister. Many children respond happily to this responsibility. However, McGovern (1982) warns that some do not.

Epilepsy not only increases the risk of disturbance among affected children, but may also have an adverse effect on the health of other family members. Mothers and siblings seem particularly at risk for increased psychiatric and psychological morbidity (Rutter et al. 1971, Hoare 1984a, Bagley 1971, Hoare, 1984b, Ferrari et al. 1983, Hoare and Kerley, 1991). Possible variables that contribute to this psychological morbidity have been explored and it has been emphasised that family members' perceptions of epilepsy are an important predictor of how they will adjust to their sibling's condition (Appolone, 1978). Other investigations of epilepsy and family adjustment have focused on parental rearing practices. These tend to be rather blame-laying, indicating parental over-protection and other restrictive practices on all family members as adversely affecting their adjustment and acceptance of the condition (Ritchie, 1981; Maj et al. 1987). Other reports have suggested that overprotective mother/child interactions can also lead to psychosocial problems for the child with epilepsy (Lothman, 1990).

Rutter et al. (1971), in an epidemiological study in the Isle of Wight, reported that one fifth of mothers of children with epilepsy had a history of a nervous breakdown, a greater incidence than that among mothers of children who had cerebral palsy or other chronic conditions. Hoare (1984a), in an examination of the extent of psychiatric disturbance in the parents and siblings of children with epilepsy, found that the rate of psychiatric disturbance was significantly greater among the siblings of children with chronic epilepsy than among siblings of children with newly diagnosed epilepsy or the general population. This implies that if a child continues to have epilepsy, it is stressful for their siblings and may adversely affect their health. Parents of the two groups of children with epilepsy were no more psychiatrically disturbed than adults in the general population. This was surprising because research by Rutter et al. (1971) had shown that the mothers of children with epilepsy have a higher rate of psychiatric disorder. Two possible explanations are the small numbers and the social-class distribution of parents: only 20% of the families in the two groups of children with epilepsy were in the lower socio-economic grouping. There was, however, a significant association between psychiatric disturbance in the child with epilepsy and increased psychiatric morbidity among mothers of children with chronic epilepsy, but not among mothers in the newly diagnosed group. This implies that the stress of coping with chronic epilepsy over a long period may adversely affect the psychological health of the mother.

Kugoh and Hosokawa (1991) have also reported higher levels of emotional distress in spouses and mothers, but not fathers of patients with epilepsy. Thompson and Upton (1992) found that 36% (n=16) of the primary-carers were considered to have severe levels of anxiety, levels which were higher than have been reported in general medical outpatients and far in excess of levels in the general population. For depression, scores were again greater than would be expected in the general population. In 23% (n=10) of cases, the primary carers were receiving treatment for psychological reasons, 11% (n=5) were receiving minor tranquillizers as an aid to sleeping, and 9% (n=4) were on antidepressants. In 36% of cases, (n=16) the primary carers were in contact with their doctor for physical complaints which included hypertension, ulcers, asthma, bronchitis, arthritis and angina.

Hoare and Kerley (1991), in a study of 108 children attending the epilepsy clinic at the Royal Hospital for Sick Children, Edinburgh, reported that there was no evidence that parents had significantly more psychiatric morbidity or a worse marital relationship than adults in the general population, as reported by Cox et al. (1987) in a previous study. However, comparison of the effects of epilepsy on family life with similar families which did not have children with epilepsy did show that the parents of children with epilepsy scored significantly higher than the comparison families on seven of the 12 measures of family stress, namely total score, dependency, cognitive impairment, restrictions for family, long-term care, anxiety about life expectancy and burden for parents. The results indicated that parents think that epilepsy imposes a burden not only for the child (increased dependency and lower intelligence), but also for the family in restricting family activities and imposing increased responsibilities for the parents. Further evidence of the stressful effects on the family was the important finding that the families of children attending special schools were under considerably more stress than those of children attending mainstream schools. These results confirm previous findings about the adverse impact of epilepsy on the family life (Bagley, 1971; Ferrari et al., 1983; Hoare, 1984a). Hoare and Kerley's (1991) analysis of maternal knowledge of and attitude toward epilepsy showed the following results: 31% (n=34) of the mothers were concerned about the possibility of death during a fit; 37% (n=40) thought their children were less intelligent than they otherwise would have been; 41% (n=44) rated their children as having reading problems; 30% (n=32) reported that their children had problems with Mathematics; 33% (n=36) said the children were more moody; 38% (n=41) reported behavioural problems; 30% (n=32) were reported to have fewer friends than siblings or peers; 54% (n=58) were thought to be less likely to obtain employment; 27% (n=29) were reported to suffer from adverse effects of drugs; more supervision was required by 32% (n=35); 34% (n=37) were regarded as presenting behaviour which was more difficult to control; 22% (n=24) of the mothers were less likely to work and 16% (n=17) reported more problems over-all for the family. The results are similar to a previous study by Hoare (1986) which found a strong association between the severity of epilepsy and maternal anxiety. The parents, particularly the mother, had a high rate of current consultation with the general medical practitioner; (42%; (n=45) of mothers and 30% (n=32) of fathers). Hoare and Kerley (1991) commented that this may be indicative of the additional burden that epilepsy imposes on the child's mother.

There was also some evidence from Hoare and Kerley's (1991) investigation that the siblings of children with epilepsy were at a greater risk of disturbance, with 25% (n=20) being rated as disturbed on the Rutter Teachers' Scale, which the authors claimed to be a more independent assessment of the child. They felt that the relatively low parental rating of 12% (n=8) disturbance among the siblings may have been an indication that the parents' attention was more focused on the child with epilepsy than on the other children. Hoare and Kerley (1991) commented that although the children in this study are not the same as an epidemiologically derived sample of all children with epilepsy living in south-east Scotland, they do represent a total population sample of children with more severe and/or longstanding epilepsy attending the only specialist out-patient service for such children in the region. Children with epilepsy who also had another serious impairment such as cerebral palsy or mental retardation do not attend that clinic. Consequently, it is claimed that the results provide an accurate account of the psychosocial adjustment of children whose main 'disability' is epilepsy.

These findings show that epilepsy can have an impact not only on the affected child but also on other members of the family. It is essential that professionals, particularly doctors and teachers who are involved with such families, are aware of the stressful effect of epilepsy on a family. They should work collaboratively towards co-ordinating a range of intervention and counselling services for both the parents and the siblings of a child with epilepsy. Such a service would provide them with opportunities to discuss any concerns or negative feelings, and help them to deal with them accordingly.

4.8 MEDICAL CONCERNS

Beech (1992) advises that family attitudes, approaches and behaviours are to some extent shaped by the degree to which family members have an informed understanding of the disorder. Clinical experience confirms that the information and knowledge that is made available to the family can be very important in the management of the child with epilepsy.

Conversely, lack of information among family members may contribute to a failure to deal with the diagnosis and provide appropriate help and support (Beech, 1992). Previous studies have reported that parents often have little knowledge about epilepsy and its treatment (Ward and Bower, 1978; Hoare 1984a; Andermann and Andermann, 1992). Pond (1981) reports that there may also be worries over management of medication, especially possible side effects. Scrambler (1994) believes that failure to consider a patient's view may contribute to non-compliance with treatment. There is also considerable patient dissatisfaction with both quantity and quality of information provided by physicians (Waizkin and Stoeckle, 1976; Boreham and Gibson, 1978; Matthews, 1983; Schneider and Conrad, 1986; Tattenborn and Kramer, 1992). There is evidence that the better educated the person with epilepsy and their carers, the fewer the associated problems (Andermann and Andermann, 1992).

Hanai (1996), in his study of quality of life in children with epilepsy found that the information communicated by physicians to 344 families before initiation of treatment was rated as "sufficiently informed" by 35% (n=120) of the total, "generally informed" by 51% (n=175) and "I think it was insufficient" by 5% (n=17). Anxieties attached to medication included a fear of side-effects such as intellectual retardation and change of personality. For currently-prescribed anti-epileptic drugs, 68% (n=234) of parents knew the name and dosage while 17% (n=58) knew the name only. Regarding treatment, 75% (n=69) of Group B (the group receiving education for disturbed children) and 60% (n=151) of Group A (the group attending mainstream classes) took their medication without failure. Twenty-eight per cent (n=71) of Group A (mainstream) forgot to take their medication several times a year, double that of the 14% (n=13) response rate of Group B (special). Seizures that were thought to occur because of irregular taking of medication were noted in 15% (n=38) of Group A (mainstream) and 34% (n=31) of Group B (special). However, 77% (n=265) of all families in the study agreed that children should regularly take medicine as prescribed by the physician. This differed significantly from the teachers' response, with only 20% (n=362) of the teachers agreeing with the statement. Ten per cent (n=181) of teachers responded that children should take adequate medicine according to the families' judgement, while none of the families agreed to this. With regard to medical concerns, 37% (n=669) of teachers wanted a closer connection between them and physicians, and 65% (n=1,178) requested guidance in the correct knowledge and treatment of seizures. The teachers also expressed concern about the lack of training and education about epilepsy in the training curriculum for school teachers.

De Boer (1995), in a survey of doctor and patient attitudes concerning communication of information in France, Germany, Italy and Spain, reported that communication between physicians and patients is not as effective as it should be and that improvement is needed. Although 70% (n=86) of physicians stated that they were prepared to provide all pertinent information, 61% (n=73) of patients said they did not have enough knowledge concerning their form of epilepsy (ranging from 83% in Spain to 38% in Germany). This discrepancy may be explained by survey sampling differences, since the German patient group was recruited from patient support groups for which ample epilepsy information is available. Patients with more severe epilepsy believed they were better informed, possibly because they see their physician more often and are therefore able to ask more questions. However, of the patient group, 35% (n=42) claimed to have received no information about epilepsy at the time of initial diagnosis. When queried about information sources, 36% (n=43) of patients said they used support groups and patient associations for information. Only 7% (n=9) of physicians believed that patients used those information sources. General physicians were considered an information source by 47% (n=58) of physicians, whereas only 15% (n=18) of patients responded that general practitioners were an information source. Of responding physicians, 46% (n=57) said they did not inform their patients about information sources. De Boer (1995) comments that the perception of information given and information received apparently differs greatly and an obvious communication gap exists.

Communication concerning drug treatment was also lacking, with 27% (n=32) of patients reporting that their physicians did not explain why a particular medicine was prescribed. This number (27%) concurred with the number of physicians who said they did not explain the medicines. Although 38% (n=46) of patients said that side effects of treatment were never mentioned, 89% (n=110) of physicians said they did inform patients about possible side effects. In summary, while physicians claim to give information about drug treatment, patients do not believe they are receiving adequate information. De Boer (1995) recommended that people with epilepsy should be better informed about their condition in order to achieve better quality of life. However, it was noted that good communication is a shared responsibility and physicians also need to be informed by their patients.

These findings have implications for paediatricians and other professionals involved in the care of children with epilepsy. For many families and teachers, epilepsy is frightening and their knowledge of the condition is often meagre. Epileptic seizures may be distressing to the child and to the parents. They may be unsure of how to cope with a child when a seizure occurs or when to call a doctor. Specific advice in these areas would increase teachers' and parents' confidence.

Effective assessment and treatment of epilepsy is dependent upon a dynamic process of mutual co-operation and sharing of information between the doctor and the individual patient or the patient's parents, in the case of younger children (The Commission for Control of Epilepsy and its Consequences, 1977; Arangio, 1980; Schneider and Conrad, 1986; Scambler and Hopkins, 1988; Zeigler, 1981). Such a process has considerable positive implications for both participants. For the physician, a knowledgeable patient is more likely to provide an accurate description of both type and frequency of seizures and potentially attain better medical compliance and assessment of effectiveness of treatment (The Commission for the Control of Epilepsy and its Consequences, 1977). The well-informed patient is not only in a position to cope with the medical implications of his or her condition but is also able to make an accurate assessment of the social, recreational and vocational limitations imposed by epilepsy and therefore minimise potential functional and emotional disturbance (Mittan, 1986; Helgeson et al., 1990; Schneider and Conrad, 1986).

The Commission for the Control of Epilepsy and its Consequences (1977) highlights the importance of patient knowledge by stating that the understanding that an individual has about any disability is related to the success the individual has in coping with the disability. Jarvie et al. (1993) state that although great advances have been made in the understanding and treatment of epilepsy, patient ignorance appears to remain high. Considerable patient ignorance has been demonstrated in regard to the purpose and results of diagnosis (Schneider and Conrad, 1986; Mittan, 1986), the causes and consequences of seizures (Mittan, 1986) and the purpose and possible side effects of medication (Mittan, 1986; Thompson and Oxley, 1989). Misunderstandings have led to restrictions in recreational activities deemed suitable for many people with epilepsy (Craig and Oxley, 1988). However, participation in social activities and gainful employment appears more closely related to positive public perceptions of disability and perceived limitations than to seizure frequency or other objective measures of epilepsy (Ryan et al., 1980; Stanley and Tillotson, 1981).

Jarvie et al. (1993) suggest that the reasons for this lack of information is the patient's (or patient's carer, in a child's case) fear and/or embarrassment and insufficient knowledge of what would be appropriate to ask, while doctors appear generally unwilling or unable to commit much time during consultations to providing medical information and answering questions to the patient's satisfaction. However, even when information is provided, patients often appear unable to comprehend or question what they have been told and what is discussed seems to be forgotten soon after consultation (Arangio, 1980; Waizkin and Stoeckle, 1976; West, 1983).

Beech (1992) constructed a 23-item questionnaire to assess awareness of basic facts about epilepsy, and suggested that it may be useful in the identification of family members whose knowledge of the condition is low and who may require appropriate counselling.

An assessment measure designed to assess general knowledge of epilepsy, the Epilepsy Knowledge Profile – General (E.K.P.-G.), was also developed by Jarvie et al. (1993). It consists of a short, self-administered questionnaire designed to assess patient's knowledge, misconceptions and fears about epilepsy. Results from the E.K.P.-G. would enable physicians to rapidly assess the overall understanding which patients and their families or carers have about epilepsy and to focus upon areas which are thought to be of specific concern or interest, e.g. poor comprehension of diagnosis and misunderstandings regarding anticonvulsant treatment. Jarvie et al. (1993) suggests that completion of the E.K.P.-G. would also provide patients with an opportunity to check their information about epilepsy, to request further information and to engage more fully in the treatment process between appointments. The questionnaire could be administered to patients attending hospital clinics or general practice surgeries as the entire process can be completed in under 10 minutes and can be scored by either trained or untrained staff. As administration and interpretation of the questionnaire does not require expert medical knowledge, the E.K.P.-G. may be applicable in a range of environments for individual or group assessment purposes. One practical application of the questionnaire could be the assessment of teachers' knowledge of the condition.

A second questionnaire, The Epilepsy Knowledge Profile – Personal (E.K.P.-P.), was also developed by Jarvie et al. (1993) and is capable of providing a rapid, yet comprehensive and valid assessment of patients' knowledge and beliefs about their own condition. While it was designed to be used in conjunction with the E.K.P.-G. to provide an extensive assessment of patient knowledge, it has been demonstrated that it can be effectively used independently. It highlights deficits in knowledge which may have a detrimental effect on seizure control and general health and safety.

4.9   CONCERNS ABOUT THE FUTURE

Pond (1981) notes that long term fears concern employability, disqualification from driving, the chances of marriage and the risks of parenthood. He adds that if the child is seriously affected, a major concern is who will look after him when family members are too old or infirm to care for them. Thompson and Upton (1992) found that parents expressed particular fears about the future with regard to who would take over the role of caring for the son or daughter when the carer becomes too old or infirm or dies. They concluded that the care of an individual with intractable epilepsy may be very stressful and the psychological ability to cope may be expected to decrease as the carers grow older and their own physical health declines. These anxieties were in keeping with those reported by Anderson and Barton (1990).

4.10   SUMMARY

This chapter examined the effect a diagnosis of epilepsy may have on the family. The findings suggest that the information given by the physicians involved in the care of the child appears to be an essential part of the family's adjustment. However, a review of the literature shows that many parents do not feel involved in a close collaboration with medical and educational professionals, nor do they receive the information they feel they need to help them understand and accept their child's condition and its possible implications. Parents clearly need to know what epilepsy is, its causes, how it is treated and followed up, the duration of treatment, its effects on schooling, what restrictions are needed and the prospects for the future. There is clearly a strong need for the relevant professionals to communicate the results of the diagnosis of epilepsy in an unambiguous, sensitive manner to parents.

As in other areas concerning epilepsy, the recurring theme is the vital importance of communication. Communication is necessary between the medical profession and parents, parents and the family and parents and the school. Professionals involved in the care of children with epilepsy should be aware of the effects on the psychological health of other members of the family, and of ways of helping the child and the family to cope with the condition. Identification of vulnerable families urgently needs much time and care, and would probably be best achieved by a team approach. Parents are likely to benefit from specific practical advice from paediatricians. Furthermore, it appears that this advice needs to be given on several occasions so that ambiguities and uncertainties can be clarified. Information and advice from associations such as Brainwave, the Irish Epilepsy Association, could complement the advice of the paediatricians or doctors. This approach is likely to enhance parents' confidence in their upbringing of the child and reduce any difficulties for the both the child and the family.

Schools, and particularly teachers, have an important role to play in helping the child with epilepsy and his parents make a successful adjustment to the problems associated with a chronic disability. The difficulties that can arise may be significantly reduced by school awareness, development of strategies for coping with seizures, acknowledgement that there may be special educational needs and planning for employment. Teachers can encourage independence and self-esteem, but if they are to do so they must be knowledgeable about epilepsy and its treatment. Paediatricians and school medical doctors can provide such information. Close liaison between doctors, Health Boards, teachers and parents is essential if the child with epilepsy and his or her family is to successfully adjust to the diagnosis and the management of the condition. Formal structural links between doctors, Schools' Medical Services, the Health Boards and parents should be established and indeed enshrined in law.

CHAPTER 5

FACTORS AFFECTING EDUCATIONAL ATTAINMENT AND SOCIAL ADJUSTMENT IN CHILDREN WITH EPILEPSY

5.1 INTRODUCTION

Besag (1994), in his review of epilepsy and education, states that misconceptions about the role of epilepsy in education abound. He stresses that the contrasting assumptions that epilepsy always has a major effect on education or that epilepsy seldom affects school performance are equally misleading. Although many children with epilepsy have no educational problems, large proportions do encounter difficulties. According to Reynolds and Trimble (1981), the exact frequency of learning problems in children with epilepsy is unknown due to difficulty in establishing prevalence rates. The figures usually quoted for children are likely to be an underestimation as they are based mainly on convulsive forms of epilepsy.

Besag (1994) believes that the long history of prejudice against children with epilepsy has led to a well-intentioned counter-reaction encouraging the attitude that all children with epilepsy are capable of coping well within the ordinary education system. He considers that the only satisfactory way of resolving the misconceptions surrounding the education of children with epilepsy is to conduct careful epidemiological studies. There have been a number of attempts to carry out such studies and Besag (1994) states that, although the details of the studies show some variability, all of them have shown unequivocally that children with epilepsy are more likely to encounter educational difficulty.

This chapter looks at a number of major international studies which have reported on the relationship between epilepsy and educational attainment among children with epilepsy. The causes of learning disabilities and behavioural disturbance, as related to epilepsy are also explored.

5.2 STUDIES OF EPILEPSY AND EDUCATIONAL ATTAINMENT

In reviewing studies of educational attainment among children with epilepsy, one must be aware of both a sampling and a definitional problem. Variation in findings may be accounted for by the fact that researchers employ different definitional criteria of epilepsy in their studies or that the samples may be biased towards children with chronic epilepsy.

Many of the earlier studies investigating the education of children with epilepsy took their samples from institutions and clinics, or tended to be over-representative of children with highly complex or atypical disorders or children from advantaged social class backgrounds whose parents sought out the more prestigious hospitals. This is well demonstrated in Bagley's (1971) study of children with epilepsy attending the neurological department at the Maida Vale Hospital, London. He reported that the average intelligence score was found to be virtually the same as that for the general population, but that the curve for intelligence was skewed to the left. This was interpreted as indicating that the sample was likely to be biased by children with neurological abnormalities or uncontrollable fits. In an American study (Needham et al., 1969), subjects were obtained from those attending welfare and private clinics. Again, Dinnage (1986) feels that this could have biased the sample towards those with greater problems, and partly accounts for the fact that the average IQ of the children with epilepsy was slightly lower than that of their siblings, although still near average. In a study of boys with epilepsy attending mainstream schools in Scotland, it was found that on a test of reasoning ability, boys with epilepsy had significantly lower scores than their classmates (Mellor and Lowitt, 1977). However, it is stated that the sample was identified through hospital and other records, and perhaps, this led to a bias towards the most severely affected children.

Understanding of epilepsy in whole communities has been greatly enhanced through community-based longitudinal studies. These include the postwar Newcastle 1000 family study (Miller et al., 1974), the Isle of Wight study of all school children on that island by Rutter et al. (1970), and the specific studies of epilepsy in children attending ordinary schools in Bedfordshire by Holdsworth and Whitmore (1974a) and in London by Kangesu et al. (1984). Other important large-scale epilepsy studies have been undertaken in Iceland (Gudmundsson, 1966), Finland (Sillanpaa, 1973), the United States (Ellenberg et al., 1985) and Italy (Pazzaglia and Frank-Pazzaglia, 1976). Although the details of the studies show some variability, all of them have shown that children with epilepsy are more likely to encounter educational difficulty.

The most complete epidemiological British national overview of epilepsy comes from the National Child Development Study (NCDS) in which the pre and postnatal histories of virtually all 17,733 children born in the week 3-9 March, 1958 in England, Scotland and Wales were documented (Ross et al., 1980). The survivors were traced to their schools at ages of seven, 11 and 16 where they were medically examined, their school performance assessed, and their parents visited by health visitors who recorded their socio-medical histories. Their subsequent progress has formed a useful basis for learning about epilepsy in unselected children.

A total of 15,496 of the original children were traced and alive at 11 years of age. It was found that 7% (n=1043) of children had a history of seizures or other episodes of loss of consciousness; 2% (n=322) or (21/1000) had a history of febrile convulsions without other epileptic problems. A further 0.3% (n=39) were reported as having epilepsy but did not fulfill the study criteria. The study's definition of epilepsy as 'recurrent paroxysmal disturbance of consciousness, sensation, or movement, primarily cerebral in origin, unassociated with acute febrile episodes', may account for the relatively low prevalence rate. A clear-cut diagnosis of non-febrile epilepsy was established in 0.4% (n=64) of children when, by the age of 11, the prevalence rate was 4.1 per 1000 on the basis of confirmatory information supplied by family doctors and paediatricians. There were slightly more boys (35) than girls (29), with an excess of fatherless children but with no bias towards any particular social class.

At age 11, 67% (n=43) of the children were in mainstream schools, 31% (n=20) were at special schools and 2% (n=1) was at home. Analysis of the educational performance of those at mainstream schools showed that non-academic tasks such as design copying were done well but that their scores in reading comprehension and mathematics tests were inferior to those of children without epilepsy. Prolonged absence from school was common; 13% (n=6) of those with epilepsy in mainstream schools and 23% (n=5) of those at special schools (excluding those in whole-time residence) missed at least one month of school in their 11th year compared with only 6% of children without epilepsy. Behavioral characteristics showed a group who were bullied as opposed to being bullies, who were meek and who showed less aggression than that noted by teachers for pupils in the study as a whole.

Of the 64 children studied at 11, 92% (n=59) took some part in the 16-year follow-up; 3% (n=2) were abroad, 2% (n=1) was a gypsy, 3% (n=2) were untraceable (Ross et al. 1983). Forty-nine per cent (n=29) had had at least one further seizure since previous contact with the study at 11, and 36% (n=21) of them had had seizures in their 16th year. Of those educated at special schools, 59% (n=13) were still having seizures in their 16th year compared with 22% (n=8) attending mainstream schools. Thirty-seven per cent (n=22) children were receiving special education, including one in a special class in a comprehensive school and 25% (n=15) were in special schools for educational backwardness (ESN (moderate) 11, ESN (severe) 4). Three per cent (n=2) were in schools for physical handicap and 7% (n=4) were in special residential schools for epilepsy. Seventeen per cent (n=10) had been formally ascertained as ESN(M) and 8% (n=5) as ESN(S). The remainder were ascertained for special education on account of epilepsy (3), deafness and physical handicap (1), physical handicap (1), ESN(M) and epilepsy (1), and physical handicap and ESN(M) (1). Epilepsy appeared to be the major handicap in four children, contrasting with educational retardation in 18. Only three of those receiving special education were regarded as having enough ability to cope with everyday reading needs such as newspapers and official forms; none were taking any public examinations.

Of the 63% (n=37) at mainstream schools, 92% (n=34) took the study's reading and Mathematics tests and achieved mean scores of 20.8 and 9.9 respectively. These were not significantly different at the 5% level from the study norms of 25.3 and 12.3. Twenty-four per cent (n=9) were taking O levels and 54% (n=20) were taking the General Certificate of Secondary Education, but their results were not available to the researchers. Twenty-four per cent (n=9) of those whose career intentions were known expected to take non-manual work and 86% (n=32) manual work. Thirty-five per cent (n=13) were considered to need sheltered accommodation and were considered unable to enter the job market.

The NCDS showed that children with epilepsy who attended special schools generally achieved poorly at school. Most were unable to get employment on leaving school. However, it is not possible to determine the precise influence of epilepsy on the achievements of the group. Ross and Tookey (1988) comment that it is probable that their performance would have been 'retarded' even if there had never been any seizures, but they do not qualify their opinion.

In the United States, Ellenberg et al. (1985) based their results on data derived from a National Collaborative Perinatal Project of the National Institute of Neurological and Communicative Disorders and Stroke (NCPP) which followed the outcome of 54,000 pregnancies in 1959. They identified 518 children who had one or more non-febrile seizures after the newborn period; 71% (n=368) of these underwent intelligence tests at seven years. Twenty-seven per cent (n=98) of children with non-febrile seizures had at least one sibling in the study. By using sibling controls, the authors concluded that, although the mean IQ score of 91.5 was less than that of the general population, it was not significantly different from that of sibling controls, thereby introducing the possibility of hereditary or genetic deficit which was independent of epilepsy. Nevertheless, their study would imply poorer intellectual performance of children with epilepsy compared with the general population.

Sillanpaa in Finland has conducted some similar epidemiological studies on epilepsy. In a recent publication, (Sillanpaa, 1992), data on 143 children with epilepsy from a population of 21,104 children aged four to 15 years was examined. The most frequent neurological impairments were mental retardation (31%; n=45), speech disorders (28%; n=39) and specific learning disorders (23%; n=33). He concluded that there was a twenty two-fold risk of the occurrence of a handicap in children with epilepsy compared with controls. In earlier reviews (Sillanpaa 1983, 1990), it was concluded that 28% of children with epilepsy did not complete their basic education or required schooling in establishments for children with learning disabilities.

A survey of Cesana, Italy, and the surrounding villages carried out by Pazzaglia and Frank-Pazzaglia (1976) identified 3% (n=38) of children with epilepsy out of a total population of 13,000 school-age children aged 6-14 years. They found a prevalence of about 3 per 1000, suggesting that they had successfully located a large proportion of the children with epilepsy. Their results reinforced the findings of earlier studies in showing a large proportion of children with educational difficulties and other problems. Of the 38 children, 71% (n=27) were of normal intelligence and 29% (n=11) were classified as 'retarded', which they defined as having an IQ of less than 80, although 91% (n=10) of the 11 children had an IQ lower than 70. They commented that 89% (n=24) of the children of normal intelligence had what they described as 'chronic depressive syndromes' with feelings of inferiority, insecurity and a tendency to give up and withdraw. About half the children had a normal record in school. Eighteen per cent (n=7) were behind their grade in school and 34% (n=13) were in special schools.

The classic Isle of Wight study (Rutter et al. 1970) found an excess of reading retardation of two years or more in almost one-fifth of the children with uncomplicated epilepsy, even if they were of average or above-average intelligence. This work is still widely quoted because it was the first true epidemiological study examining all children around ten years of age in a defined geographical location.

Gastaut (1965), using comprehensive psychological testing on children with epilepsy in Britain, showed that as many as a third had perceptual difficulties which could cause a considerable handicap in learning to read and write.

Stores and Hart (1976) examined reading skills in children aged seven to 14 years with generalised epileptiform discharges and focal discharges attending mainstream schools in England. Seventeen children (ten boys and seven girls) with electrographically generalised discharges were matched for age and sex with seventeen children who had persistent focal discharges in either temporal lobe or the immediate adjacent area. Each child was then matched for age and sex with a child who did not have epilepsy. Their conclusions were as follows:

1. The reading skills of children with electrographically generalised epilepsy and subclinical seizure discharges (occurring to the extent usually seen in childhood epilepsy of this type) appeared to be no worse than those of matched controls who did not have epilepsy.
2. In contrast, children with persistent focal spike discharges, especially if located in the left hemisphere dominant for speech, tended to have lower reading levels than their matched controls without epilepsy, especially in the case of reading accuracy.
3. The inferior performance of the focal group as a whole was largely attributable to those children with left hemisphere focal spikes, and these were predominantly boys.
4. The reading skills of boys with epilepsy, whatever their type of epilepsy, were inferior to those of girls with epilepsy; this sex difference was not seen in the control children who did not have epilepsy.
5. The long-term use of the drug phenytoin was associated with lower levels of reading skill than were other forms of anti-epileptic medication.

Glowinski (1973) has also produced evidence to suggest that patients with temporal lobe epilepsy find it more difficult to remember meaningful verbal material than other types of material. Other authors have reported findings at variance with the above. Camfield et al. (1984) were unable to show any difference on cognitive testing between children with left and right temporal lobe foci. Giordani et al. (1985) found that overall intelligence was the same in children and young adults with generalised and with partial seizures, but that those with primarily or secondarily generalised seizures obtained significantly lower scores on tests related to attention, visuospatial orientation and sequencing ability. However, Seidenberg et al. (1986) did not find the site of the EEG focus to be significant in their test results.

Holdsworth and Whitmore's (1974a) study was not based on an entire childhood population because it excluded children attending special schools. Eighty-five children with epilepsy in a rural community in England fulfilled the experimental criteria of attendance at a mainstream school and having had a seizure during the prior twelve months (52 children), or being treated with antiepileptic drugs over that period (33 children). The relatively low prevalence figures obtained by the study, namely 1.6 per 1000 in the primary schools and 2.4 per 1000 in the secondary schools, probably reflect the fact that additional cases were excluded because they were not attending mainstream schools. Sixty-four of the children were classified into three groups, based on their educational performance. Thirty-one per cent (n=20) were found to be maintaining an average to superior level of performance, 53% (n=34) were 'holding their own at a below-average level' and 16% (n=10) were seriously behind. They found that barely one-third of the children sampled were making wholly satisfactory progress; half the children were achieving a very indifferent performance in the classroom (holding their own at a below-average level); one in six was falling appreciably behind in work, and one in five had behavioural problems. The authors emphasised that even in mainstream schools, children with epilepsy are an educationally vulnerable group. The children were described as having good rates of attendance – only ten (seven of whom were boys) were reported to have poor rates of attendance. They felt that the data did not suggest that poor school attendance might have contributed to the large proportion of boys among the educationally retarded. Rutter et al. (1970) observe in this connection that poor school attendance is not the only factor contributing to educational failure, since among children with normal intelligence and normal rates of attendance there still tends to be an increased rate of reading retardation. Holdsworth and Whitmore (1974a) were not able to investigate why these children were absent so often from school, but recurrent seizures were not the main factor, since frequent seizures were no more common among the children with poor attendance than among those with good or average attendance. The frequency of seizures and their occurrence during the previous twelve months or in school seemed to have no bearing on educational outcome or poor attendance. In fact the only child in the survey with daily (petit mal) seizures was in Group A which consisted of those children who were maintaining an average to superior general level of performance. The effect of the type of seizure was less certain. Three of the four children with petit mal alone were in Group A and none were in Group C, which consisted of those who had fallen seriously behind. Of the children who had major seizures and were classified as 'educationally retarded', barely one-quarter were in Group A and 18% were in Group C. Furthermore, almost all the 'educationally retarded' children were subject to major epilepsy, and only one had petit mal alone, a significant difference compared with the most successful children. The teaching staff were also asked to assess attentiveness and behaviour, and 42% (n=27) of the children were noted to have problems with attention and were described in terms such as listless, lethargic, dull, apathetic and 'just not with us'. Absence seizures were unlikely to account for the descriptions since only five children had these.

Holdsworth and Whitmore (1971), in an earlier study of primary children with epilepsy attending mainstream schools, found that 42% of the pupils were described by their teachers as being 'markedly inattentive'. The children were described as lethargic, absent-minded, sleepy, doped, lacking in concentration or otherwise unresponsive to some extent to what was happening in class. Inattentiveness was found to be associated with unsatisfactory educational progress.

Stores et al. (1978), examining inattentiveness in 36 boys and 35 girls with epilepsy attending mainstream schools, found that according to their teachers and parents, the boys were significantly more inattentive and overactive than the girls. They performed significantly less well on tests of sustained attention and perceptual accuracy. No such sex difference was seen in any of the measures among children who did not have epilepsy. The results were of particular interest with regard to the distractibility test. Whereas experimentally increased classroom noise lowered the scores of the children who did not have epilepsy, such increases improved the performance of the children who had epilepsy, suggesting that these children were in some way under-aroused and derived benefit from the alerting effect of the noise.

Stedman et al. (1982) found that among the children with epilepsy attending mainstream schools in the Oxford region, only 15% could be considered as making fairly satisfactory school progress, and nearly half were more than two years behind in reading, spelling or mathematics. It was noted that boys were more retarded in reading than girls. The authors recommended that there should be more communication between doctors and teachers, so that teachers realise which of their pupils have epilepsy and devise special teaching programmes to meet their needs.

In studies in the U.S.A., Seidenberg et al. (1986) found that, as a group, children with epilepsy were making less academic progress than expected for their age and IQ level. Academic deficiencies were greatest in mathematics, followed by spelling, reading, comprehension and word recognition. In the study by Ounsted et al. (1966), a high proportion of the children with temporal lobe epilepsy were also found to have made poor academic attainments despite average or above average levels of general intelligence. Giordani et al. (1985), found that general intelligence was the same in children and young adults with generalised and with partial seizures, but that those with primarily or secondarily generalised seizures performed significantly less well on tests related to attention, visuospatial orientation and sequencing ability.

Schuler et al. (1997) analysed the school performance and the social integration of children with epilepsy, aged between six and sixteen years, with normal psychomotor development attending mainstream Swiss schools. Their siblings who did not have epilepsy and were also attending mainstream schools were used as a control group. It was found that the children with epilepsy had significantly poorer school performance, more concentration problems (53% vs 6%), less self-confidence (17% vs 4%), more relationship problems (35% vs 19%), and more school failures (30% vs 5%). No differences between the two groups were found concerning school absenteeism.

The results of these studies raise some pertinent questions, both with regard to additional input for children attending mainstream schooling and in relation to the provision in the special schools for children with epilepsy. The consensus from these studies is that, although the educational progress of some children with epilepsy is in the normal or superior range, a large proportion has a degree of educational difficulty. Areas in which difficulties are experienced tend to be reading, spelling and mathematics. Inattentiveness and concentration difficulties among children with epilepsy also affect educational progress. An understanding of the problems that might arise might facilitate early intervention and the possibility of minimising any subsequent disruption to the child's education.

5.3 CAUSES OF LEARNING DISABILITIES AND BEHAVIOURAL DISTURBANCE AMONG CHILDREN WITH EPILEPSY

There are many possible causes for learning disability and behavioural disturbance in a child with epilepsy. Besag (1994) summarises the factors that may affect learning and behaviour as follows:

5.3.1 The Epilepsy Itself
Prodrome
Prodrome is the period of hours or days before a seizure, or cluster of seizures, during which the child may experience various symptoms, including irritability or general dullness. These symptoms resolve with the seizure. Parents often recognise the prodrome and may comment that the child is "working up to a seizure", adding that they cannot wait for the seizure to occur because they know that their child will be all right again when it does. Besag (1994) advises that the mood changes associated with the prodrome may affect both behaviour and learning. He warns that punishment of the child's poorer performance by teachers or others may add to the burden, lowering the child's self-esteem and increasing the likelihood of behaviour change. It would be quite inappropriate for the teacher to admonish or punish the child for being mildly irritable during this period. Although the need for discipline remains, the way in which it is administered needs to be moderated at this time.

Aura
The aura is often described as being the warning of the seizure. It is in fact a simple partial seizure, although it may herald a more widely spread abnormal discharge leading to a complex partial seizure or generalized seizure in many cases. The aura typically lasts for a few seconds but it may be perceived as lasting longer because of subjective distortions of time. There are many varieties, but the classical auras are unpleasant sensations in the epigastrium, odd smells or flashing lights. Children experiencing multiple auras may find these much more distressing than full-blown seizures, since auras occur in full consciousness and are usually remembered. The child may think that this is a sign of madness and may be unwilling to tell others of the experience. Auras may result in both anxiety and behavioural change because they usually herald full-blown seizures. According to Besag (1994), all of these factors are likely to lead to problems if auras occur in the classroom, particularly if teachers do not understand why the child appears distressed and adopt a punitive approach. They may also occur many times a day, adding greatly to the distress they cause.

Automatism
Fenton (1972) defined an automatism as a state of clouding of consciousness which occurs during or immediately after a seizure, and during which the individual retains control of posture and muscle tone but performs simple or complex movements and actions without being aware of what is happening. Automatisms occurring after an obvious tonic-clonic seizure may be more readily accepted than those occurring as a result of a complex partial seizure, since the latter may not be recognized as being a seizure at all. Besag (1994) emphasises that they may also have profound educational implications as they can sometimes appear quite bizarre and may easily be misinterpreted by teachers or classmates. He warns that teasing or rejection at school is quite likely to occur unless the situation is managed well.

Post-Ictal Changes
After a seizure, depending on the parts of the brain involved and the duration, various changes may occur. Sleepiness is the most common post-ictal change. If a child needs to sleep for long periods after a seizure this may be very disruptive to schooling (Besag, 1994). Other common features include confusion, aggression, concentration difficulties, depressive, manic and schizophreniform paranoid problems. Between these extremes, various degrees of irritability and confusion may occur. Such changes are usually short-lived and do not necessarily require treatment, but certainly require appropriate support and understanding. These difficulties can be recognised and easily managed by trained staff, but may be regarded as disruptive behaviour by teachers or staff

inexperienced in epilepsy, leading to further problems in school (Aldenkamp et al.1990; Besag, 1988).

Inter-Ictal Psychoses
They are not usually seen in children but do occur in adolescents and adults. They may be either manic or schizophreniform, and may last for several months. Besag (1994) emphasises that if they are prolonged or severe, they impair education to a major degree until they resolve or are treated satisfactorily.

Focal Discharges
The aura already described is a type of focal discharge, but one that is short-lived. Frequent focal discharges may result in several different changes, depending on the location of the disturbance in the brain. The literature contains reports of an association between left-sided temporal discharges and aggressive behaviour in young men. Stores et al. (1978) emphasised the association between deficits in reading skills and focal spike discharges in either the left temporal lobe or the immediate adjacent area. Besag (1995) also says that his experience suggests that frequent frontal discharges may affect behaviour and learning to a major degree. He stresses the importance of carefully planned EEG investigation of children who may have abnormal EEG discharges and who are failing educationally.

Type and Frequency of Seizures
The occurrence of frequent seizures can lead to considerable life disruption for a child, particularly in relation to school (Dodrill, 1986; Reiner, 1982). Many teachers find it difficult to cope with seizures and this may result in the child returning home after even a brief seizure for which a short rest is adequate (Brainwave, the Irish Epilepsy Association, 1991). This can lead to considerable loss of time in school with associated educational difficulties, particularly if the child is experiencing daily or even weekly seizures (Besag, 1987; Besag, 1988).

According to Besag (1994), absence seizures interrupt awareness and, if they occur frequently, may make learning and socialisation very difficult. Although most children with occasional typical absence seizures progress well, some who have very frequent absence seizures may encounter considerable difficulties. He warns that in the small number of children who have such frequent epileptiform discharges, educational progress and social interaction are clearly hampered to a major degree. Although the manifestations of the discharges may vary widely from one child to another, Besag (1994) warns that it seems that impairment of educational awareness and performance while they are occurring, is inevitable. Some children respond by exhibiting withdrawn behaviour. Those who enter bouts of nonconvulsive status epilepticus, when the subtle seizures are so frequent that the child does not recover fully between them, may exhibit highly disturbed behaviour when they emerge from these states.

Many children with recurrent seizures experience unpredictable patterns in terms of seizure frequency. They may experience a number of weeks in which they are seizure free, followed by a cluster of seizures together, which may impair their cognitive abilities at the time. Brainwave, the Irish Epilepsy Association (1991) advocates a special educational programme to deal with this situation. Such children may be inappropriately placed in schools for the mentally handicapped or may have no educational facility available to them (Besag, 1988).

Injury Due to Seizures:
Some types of seizures can result in significant injury, particularly if appropriate medical care is not readily available. Some seizure conditions may also be life-threatening as in the case of status epilepticus where the child experiences one seizure after another without regaining consciousness. For such children it is essential that experienced personnel and medical facilities are available to treat the situation promptly, thus preventing brain damage or death (Brainwave, the Irish Epilepsy Association, 1991).

Seizures Which Are Difficult to Recognise
Many children experience significant problems at school because of the occurrence of seizures which are difficult to recognise. These may include brief absences which may be interpreted as lack

of co-operation, inattentiveness or at times, disruptive behaviour. Likewise, complex partial seizures, particularly of frontal lobe origin, can be very difficult both to recognise and diagnose. Brainwave, the Irish Epilepsy Association (1991) advises that the availability of a detailed assessment for such cases could help alleviate the significant disruption associated with such seizures and may allow the child to return to mainstream education successfully.

As shown, the various causes of learning disabilities and behavioural disturbance in a child with epilepsy are wide-ranging. Besag (1994) warns that the educational implications of the epilepsy itself can have a profound effect on both the child's behaviour and educational progress. If the child's educational needs are to be fulfilled successfully, the professionals involved in their education require comprehensive knowledge of these factors. In situations where children experience unpredictable seizure frequency, behaviour and cognitive abilities may be affected and provision of a special educational programme, as advocated
by Brainwave, the Irish Epilepsy Association (1991), may be required.

5.3.2   Treatment of the Epilepsy
Parents and teachers often worry that anti-epileptic medication will impair a child's performance at school. Although this concern is not always justified, it is undoubtedly true that anti-epileptic drugs (AEDS) may have adverse effects on both cognitive function and behaviour (Reynolds and Trimble, 1981; O'Donohue, 1994).

Phenobarbitone, Primidone (Mysoline) and the Benzodiazepines
Phenobarbitone, primidone and benzodiazepines are particularly notorious for their adverse effects on childhood behaviour and have often been causally implicated in the learning difficulties of children with epilepsy (O'Donohue, 1994). According to O'Donohue (1994), phenobarbitone may have a dulling effect on attention and perception resulting in inability to maintain vigilance over long periods of time.

Hutt et al. (1968) found that phenobarbitone had an adverse effect on intellectual tasks involving sustained effort and attention. Vinning (1987) compared phenobarbitone and valproic acid with reference to their effects on cognition and behaviour in children being treated for epilepsy and found that phenobarbitone produced more adverse side-effects. Brent et al. (1990) have reported that phenobarbitone increases the risk of major depressive illness in children with epilepsy.
In the National Child Development Study in the United Kingdom, it was found that phenobarbitone was prescribed to 90% (n=58) of children but 56% (n=36) had their treatment changed to phenytoin, usually because of the side-effects rather than because of its failure to control seizures (Ross et al., 1980).

An investigation of the long-term course of intelligence and cognitive skills in children with epilepsy by Bourgeois et al. (1983) found that drug toxicity (especially of phenobarbitone) predicted an IQ decrease more definitively than other factors. The authors suggest that total seizure control, especially in young children, should not be achieved at the price of repeated episodes of drug toxicity.

Chen et al. (1996) compared the cognitive effects of carbamazepine, phenobarbitaone and sodium valporate in children with newly diagnosed epilepsy. No difference in the IQ or Bender-Gestalt scores were found between the groups, but auditory-evoked potentials were increased in children receiving phenobarbitone, suggesting that it may affect cortical functioning.

A surprising finding of the study carried out by Holdsworth and Whitmore (1974a) was the statistically significant result that children whose behaviour was not causing concern were twice as likely to be taking phenobarbitone.

Primidone can sometimes produce alarming personality changes ('mysoline madness') and the EEG can be useful in distinguishing this from a consequence of a deterioration in the patient's epileptic state (O' Donohue, 1994).

Phenytoin (Epanutin)
O' Donohue (1994) has reported that chronic intoxication with phenytoin can lead to intellectual deterioration. Stores and Hart (1976), in a study of factors associated with the progress of children with epilepsy attending normal schools, found that the reading skills of those children who had taken phenytoin for at least two years were significantly inferior to those who had taken other anti-epileptic drugs over a similar period.

Andrews et al. (1986) found that phenytoin particularly affected tasks involving short-term memory. Vinning (1987) also mentioned its adverse effects on attention, problem solving ability and performance of visuomotor tasks.

Thompson et al. (1981) also found that the subjects' performance was significantly poorer on two tests of memory, one of concentration, two of decision-making speed, and one of motor speed. A significant number of subjects described themselves as feeling fatigued. The authors concluded that the possible detrimental effects of phenytoin are of considerable importance and that other drugs should be considered.

Ethosuximide (Zarontin)
O' Donohue (1994) reports that ethosuximide has been linked occasionally with adverse effects on learning in children, mainly as a cause of global mental impairment. A combination of ethosuximide and barbiturate was reported by Guey et al. (1967) to have deleterious effects on concentration as well as on performance on a variety of verbal and non-verbal tasks. Their study illustrates the need to monitor blood levels and to consider interactions when investigating anticonvulsant actions.

However, Browne (1983) has shown that the psychosocial effects of ethosuximide are minimal while its effectiveness in reducing absences and spike-wave EEG discharges greatly improves intellectual function, behaviour and school-performance.

Sodium Valproate (Epilim)
Sodium valproate is much less detrimental to cognitive function than either phenytoin or phenobarbitone, and such side effects as have been recorded appeared to be dose-related (Trimble and Thompson, 1984).

Behavioural changes, including irritability, hyperactivity, lassitude and drowsiness seem to be related to high levels of sodium valproate (Herranz et al. 1982). Drowsiness is rarely experienced with sodium valproate alone but may occur if the drug is added to phenobarbitone (O'Donohue, 1994).

Clonazepam (Rivotril)
Trimble (1988) reports that clonazepam (CZP) and phenobarbital (PB) may be associated with gross overactivity, severe behavioural change and cognitive impairment, but clobazam is less likely to have these effects.

Carbamazepine (Tegretol)
Since its introduction, reports on the effect of carbamazepine on both cognitive function and behaviour have been consistently favourable. An important advantage of carbamazepine compared with phenobarbitone and phenytoin is that it does not seem to impair cognitive function during long-term administration (O'Donohue, 1994).

Thompson and Trimble (1983) showed that, in patients who had been given psychological testing using a battery of tests which included memory, attention and concentration, perceptual speed, decision-making speed and motor speed tasks, those on monotherapy with either phenytoin or sodium valproate had impairments in performance at high serum levels which were approximately twice those observed at low serum levels of the drugs, even though both high and low serum level were within the therapeutic ranges for the drugs. In contrast, carbamazepine-treated patients showed minimal changes in performance during both high and low serum levels (Thompson and Trimble, 1983). Furthermore, there is considerable evidence that carbamazepine is psychotropic in its effects, while phenobarbitone, and perhaps other drugs also, may sometimes exacerbate or even precipitate affective disturbances in adults and children (Trimble, 1988; Brent et al., 1990).

Vigabatrin (Sabril) and Lamotrigine (Lamictal)
The effects of the newer drugs, vigabatrin and lamotrigine, on cognition and behaviour, have not yet been fully assessed. However, vigabatrin has been reported as causing sedation and memory problems in a small proportion of patients (Remy and Beaumont, 1989). Trimble (1988) has reported that vigabatrin (VGB) can be associated with gross behavioural change in older children being treated for partial seizures.

Stores (1975) reviewed the possible effects of anti-epileptic drugs on the learning process and emphasised that there is a widespread belief among teachers that children treated with these drugs are inevitably 'handicapped'. The author did not define what this meant exactly. He also considered that this belief contributes to the under-expectations which teachers generally have about children with epilepsy.

Other studies have failed to show significant effect of anti-epileptic drugs on cognitive functioning (Dodrill and Temkin 1989, Meador et al., 1990). Aldenkamp et al., (1993), studying the effects of withdrawal of anti-epileptic medication, attributed differences in cognitive functioning between the subjects to their underlying seizure condition rather than to the effects of withdrawing from the anti-epileptic drugs. No significant improvement was noted after withdrawal of anti-epileptic drugs, suggesting limited impact on higher order cognitive functioning.

O'Donohue (1994) emphasises that the effects on cognitive function of anti-epileptic drugs are greatly amplified by their administration in polytherapy regimes. He advises that drug-related cognitive dysfunction may often be reversed simply by changing to monotherapy, and such a change also facilitates more reliable monitoring of serum drug levels, an essential investigation in any child with behaviour and/or learning problems who is receiving medication for epilepsy (Stores, 1975; Vinning, 1987).

Literature on the effects of anti-epileptic medication on both cognitive function and behaviour shows that they undoubtedly affect the children. Reported side effects include: headaches, memory difficulties, tiredness and drowsiness, lack of concentration, disruptive behaviour, hyperactivity, tantrums, weight gain, skin problems, dizziness and visual disturbance and intellectual deterioration. The educational implications of these side effects can be quite profound and it is of utmost importance that educators of children with epilepsy are aware of them and are trained to deal with them.

5.3.3 Reactions to the Epilepsy
O'Donohue (1994) states that quite apart from the effects of structural brain abnormality, seizure discharges and drugs on attention and learning ability in the child with epilepsy, it seems likely that unfavourable environmental factors at home and at school may adversely affect the development of the child's cognitive and social skills. Hartlage and Green (1972) suggested that the academic achievement of the child with epilepsy may be more closely related to environmental factors than to any specific disability of neurological origin. In their study they found that the academic and social underachievement of children with epilepsy could be attributed, at least in part, to inappropriate dependency on their parents. They did not feel that this overdependency was due to any single faulty attitude on the part of the parent (such as overprotectiveness), but rather to the direct impact of epilepsy and its treatment on the child's psychological development causing a delay in emotional growth. However, overprotection or rejection by the parents and other authority figures may influence behaviour of children with epilepsy to a major degree (Besag, 1995).

Both teachers and parents often believe that a child with epilepsy is intrinsically incapable of doing as well academically as unaffected children. Bagley (1971) reported that teachers tended to under-estimate the intellectual potential of children with epilepsy, basing their estimates on attainment levels that were often below their true ability. Low attainment may therefore be partly attributable to the effects of under-expectation and lack of stimulation.

The child with epilepsy may well face similarly inappropriate and unhelpful attitudes at school from teachers and other children. Teachers may harbour misconceptions about epilepsy in the absence of adequate instruction in their training courses. Again unnecessary restrictions may be imposed and recreational and other school activities curtailed on the assumption that physical or mental exertion may be harmful. The child can become a social outcast in the process, and may face ridicule or hostility from other children (Stores, 1981).

Besag (1995) states that restrictions imposed by teachers or teasing by other pupils at school can have a profound effect on the child's feelings of self-esteem and, consequently, on their behaviour. A particularly noteworthy finding of the Pazzaglia and Frank-Pazzaglia study (1976) was the unsatisfactory attitudes of teachers and parents and of other pupils in the class. The teachers felt that they had no training to deal with epilepsy, and most were unwilling to teach pupils with epilepsy; 5% (n=2) of the teachers thought that all pupils with epilepsy should be taught in special classes. They also reported that the reactions of other pupils and their parents to pupils with epilepsy were very unfavourable if the child had seizures at school. Both over-protection and rejection can be very damaging to the child, both in terms of personal and educational progress (Besag, 1995).

Holdsworth and Whitmore (1974b), in a study of the attitudes of teachers towards children with epilepsy attending mainstream schools, found that although teachers were more sympathetic to pupils with epilepsy, some teachers had lower expectations for their work. This, in turn, led to underachievement by the children.

5.3.4 Associated Brain Damage
Besag (1995) reports that most children with epilepsy do not have brain damage, but epilepsy may either be caused by brain damage or, more rarely, may cause it, particularly if prolonged seizures occur. In either case, the brain damage itself may be the cause of behavioural disturbance; e.g., frontal lobe damage may cause gross disinhibition, and brain damage elsewhere may result in cognitive or motor deficits which may be frustrating for the child. It is very important that careful, periodic, psychometric assessments are carried out to determine the educational strengths and needs of the child experiencing educational difficulty.

5.3.5 Causes Equally Applicable To Those Without Epilepsy
Besag (1995) stresses that educational difficulties can have a large number of causes, and the child with epilepsy is subject to all the usual ones. The fact that he or she is having educational difficulties does not necessarily mean the epilepsy is to blame. Behavioural problems in a child with epilepsy may be quite unrelated to the medical condition. A child with epilepsy may have behavioural disturbance for all the reasons that children without epilepsy have disturbed behaviour. It is important that the behavioural problems are viewed in the context of the child's life situation so that epilepsy is not blamed for causes which are quite unrelated to the medical condition.

Although it has been reported by Rutter et al. (1970) and Holdsworth and Whitmore (1971) that poor school attendance was not a contributory factor to the problems of school children with epilepsy, it may undoubtedly become a problem if children are frequently withheld from school or often sent home after an attack by over-cautious parents or teachers. In general, it is sufficient for the child to lie down to quietly recover from a seizure, and then allow him to continue with normal school activities, rather than treat each seizure as an emergency (Stores, 1981).

5.4   SUMMARY
This chapter examined the factors affecting educational attainment and social adjustment in children with epilepsy. Review of studies of epilepsy and educational attainment show that a large proportion of children with epilepsy has a degree of educational difficulty.

Possible effects on learning and behaviour are among the major concerns expressed regarding children with epilepsy. Besag (1995) believes that learning difficulties, whether they occur as a result of the epilepsy or of other causes, may not only affect behaviour but can significantly influence the future prospects of the child. O'Donohue (1994) stresses that since it seems likely that cognitive defects may generate disturbed behaviour in children with epilepsy, early recognition and treatment of these deficits may produce beneficial results, both in the learning situation and in the personality development of the child. From the literature it appears that there may be many different factors connected with the causation of learning difficulties in children with epilepsy. Determining the causes of learning and behavioural problems and intervening to prevent or minimise the disadvantage to the child are key aspects of management of children with epilepsy who are experiencing difficulties at school.

The educational difficulties experienced by children with epilepsy and the factors influencing their progress should be an integral part of existing preservice teacher training courses. The Teacher Unions, as part of in-service provision for teachers who are already trained, should also provide courses for teachers who are already trained. Such programmes should serve to heighten teacher awareness of the possible educational and medical difficulties encountered by many children with epilepsy. They should also be specifically directed towards informing teachers as to how best to maximise instructional and educational opportunities for the child with epilepsy.

CHAPTER SIX

EDUCATIONAL LEGISLATION AND PROVISION FOR CHILDREN WITH EPILEPSY IN ENGLAND AND IRELAND

6.1 INTRODUCTION

Besag (1987) states that the concept of segregating people simply on the basis of their having a disease or disorder is no longer either accepted or acceptable. At various times in the past the leper colony, the mental asylum and the TB sanatorium were considered to be not only acceptable, but also desirable places for people with epilepsy. According to Besag (1987), the purpose of these institutions was sometimes not so much to offer a service to those with the condition as to segregate them from society, sparing the general public the inconvenience or perceived risk of having them in the community. Although Hippocrates (450 BC) tried to dispel the attitude that epilepsy was the result of possession by evil spirits, the feeling that epilepsy might be a bad influence on others or might even be infectious continued through the centuries. These beliefs and attitudes have been explored in Chapter 2. Gradually, the kindlier elements of society provided centres where people with epilepsy could escape from a hostile world intolerant of their condition (Grant, 1981). Today with the move towards integrated education few epilepsy centres remain in Europe, but those that do provide a much-needed service for children with difficult epilepsy.

This chapter looks at the historical development of the epilepsy centres in England and other countries, and their present-day role in provision for people with epilepsy. The reasons for referral to schools for children with epilepsy are also examined. Educational legislation in England and Wales is briefly outlined. The English system of education is used for comparative purposes because the Irish and English education systems have developed in parallel and from similar orgins, and because the structures are similar. Moreover, special needs education in Northern Ireland is very similar to that which applies in the United Kingdom generally, and the English system of education, particularly with regard to provision for children with epilepsy, is considerably more developed. The final section provides a critique of educational legislation and provision for children with epilepsy in the Republic of Ireland.

6.2 HISTORICAL BACKGROUND OF EPILEPSY CENTRES

One of the earliest recorded establishments with a more caring attitude to epilepsy was founded at the end of the 15th century, when the monks at the Priory of Saint Valentine at Rufach, in Alsace provided a 'hospice for epileptics'. In 1773, the Bishop of Wurzburg established a home for people with epilepsy. By the 19th century, the practice of putting the insane in chains was discontinued, and because people with epilepsy had often been confined with the insane, this was of benefit to them also (Grant, 1981). In general, it was only from the time of Pinel (1745-1826) in France, and the Tukes in England that people with epilepsy confined to institutions became the object of systematic medical attention (Temkin, 1971).

In 1815, Esquirol, a 19th century physician, made a strong plea for the establishment of special provisions for people with epilepsy. However, this was because he thought that the sight of an epileptic attack might be sufficient to make a healthy person develop epilepsy (Grant, 1981). About 1850 it became the practice in England to confine patients with epilepsy to separate wards in lunatic asylums. When this kind of segregation became established the logical outcome was a demand for special institutions for people with epilepsy.

This demand began to be fulfilled from 1860, when the National Hospital for the Paralysed and Epileptic was opened in Queen Square, London. In Germany, in 1867, four people with epilepsy were taken into custodial care in a farmhouse outside the town of Bielfield by a Lutheran pastor. One of the most influential epilepsy centres was established in that farmhouse when, in 1872, Pastor Friedrich von Bovelschwingh took over what became the famous Bethel Centre. Subsequently, in 1882, the colony at 'Meer en Bosch', in Heemstede, the Netherlands and the

Filadelfia colony at Dianalund in Denmark were founded. Based on the Bethel experience, several centres in the United Kingdom opened, including the first special institution for people with epilepsy at Maghull, near Liverpool. The Chalfont Centre for Epileptics in Buckinghamshire followed this in 1894. The centre at Lingfield, now known as St. Piers Lingfield Hospital School, was established in 1898, and the David Lewis Epileptic Colony, Cheshire was opened in 1904. These three centres remain and, together with the Park Hospital in Oxford, form the nucleus for intensive work with people who have difficult epilepsy.

Meanwhile, progress was being made elsewhere, particularly in Europe and the United States of America where similar developments were taking place. 'Colonies' or residential centres for persons with epilepsy were founded initially at Gallipolis, Ohio, in 1891, followed by a colony at Sonyea, New York State. Ultimately by 1933, 14 institutions were developed in various states, but most of these did not survive. In France, a day hospital specifically for epileptic patients was established at Creteil, near Paris. In the Netherlands, outpatient clinics and special centres for epilepsy had been established in nine locations (Meinardi, 1972). In Norway, a country which had never had epileptic centres, a bill was passed in Parliament in 1970-1971 for further development of the care of patients with epilepsy, based on the developments in Britain (Henriksen, 1972). Until then there had been one National Hospital for Epileptics, the Statens Sykehus for Epileptics at Sandvika. The National Centre for Epilepsy in Sandvika in Norway continues to provide a centre for research and assessment. In Denmark, the Filadelfia Colony remains functional at Dianalund, and the Danish Epilepsy Association has founded a day centre for severely handicapped people with epilepsy in a suburb of Copenhagen (Lund and Randrup, 1972).

Many colonies or centres for persons with epilepsy evolved in many parts of the world between the middle of the 19th and early 20th century. According to Grant (1981) they developed to provide a haven of retreat from an increasingly industrialised and hostile world, and were originally intended to provide custodial care for many years or for life. They were largely self-supporting communities and it is significant that many of the centres in Britain, Europe and the USA were deliberately established away from the urban areas of industry and employment. Grant (1981) believes that they provided a much-needed service that most of society had neglected. However, by the middle of this century, a new role for the epilepsy centres was necessary.

6.3 THE PRESENT ROLE OF THE EPILEPSY CENTRES

There are currently three residential schools specialising in the treatment of epilepsy in England. Children who attend these schools have severe epilepsy and/or educational failure. Besag (1988) states that most children with epilepsy will attend mainstream schools, but an important minority require additional educational provision, and a few can only have their special educational needs satisfactorily fulfilled in a residential establishment with particular experience in the management of epilepsy. Students are referred to residential special schools for children with epilepsy because of problems which they can experience. Such problems can include: frequent seizures, injury in seizure, risk of status epilepticus, variable seizure frequency, post-ictal problems, anti-epileptic drug problems, inadequate control and difficult-to-recognise epilepsy. The possible reasons for referral to a residential epilepsy special school as summarised by Besag (1987, 1988b), are given as follows:

Difficult Epilepsy

Frequent seizures: If seizures occur frequently, or if they tend to 'cluster', occurring in intermittent bursts, schooling can become very disrupted. Frequent major seizures are likely to be a cause of disruption, both to the sufferer and to the other students in the class. Besag (1988) comments that regrettably some teachers, inexperienced in epilepsy, are terrified of seizures and are unwilling or unable to cope with children who have frequent seizures. In a residential environment where teachers are trained in the management of seizures, both the teacher and the other students can deal with the situation with the minimum of disruption to the teaching programme. Advice and back up from on-site medical and nursing staff are readily available, if required. In the epilepsy special school, the child spends the minimum period of time out of the educational situation. Because the teachers know that medical care is immediately at hand, they are prepared to take the child back soon after a seizure, even if the seizure has been severe or if there is a possibility of further seizures.

Frequent 'absences' and other forms of subtle seizures require a specialised teaching technique. The teacher needs to be trained to recognise these attacks and to repeat what has been said, sometimes several times, until the child is fully aware and able to assimilate the material. If the seizure frequency is variable the teachers can monitor the situation and can vary the amount of work they aim to cover, giving more in the good phases and making allowances in the bad phase.

Injury in seizures: The atonic drop attack is notorious for causing severe injury because the child falls to the ground without any warning. Although she/he will usually recover consciousness immediately, s/he may require treatment for the injuries sustained. Severe injury may also result from tonic seizures when the child stiffens, and the head may fall in a long arc to the ground. A significant number of children also injure themselves in generalised tonic clonic or clonic seizures. Occasionally, injury may also occur in massive myoclonic jerks. With on-site medical and nursing care, the child can be assessed, treated as necessary, and returned to the classroom with the minimum of delay. Head injury observations can be continued overnight, if they are considered to be necessary. Teachers can understandably become anxious if a child frequently injures himself in seizures unless they know that medical care, advice and treatment are readily available.

Risk of status epilepticus: Status epilepticus may be defined as repeated seizures without recovery of consciousness or a prolonged seizure lasting twenty minutes or longer. According to Besag (1988) it is a medical emergency because permanent brain damage can result, particularly in young children, if it is not treated promptly. He states that even if a child is subject only to infrequent seizures it may be justifiable to educate him in a residential establishment capable of providing rapid emergency treatment where bouts of status epilepticus are experienced from time to time.

Variable seizure frequency: Some children can remain free of seizures for a few weeks or months and then have frequent seizures over a similar period. In the residential special school, allowances can be made for gaps in the educational programme during the bad phases and additional medical treatment given if necessary. During the good phases, additional teaching can be provided to help the student catch up.

Post-ictal problems: After a seizure, the common post-ictal manifestation is sleepiness. Some children, however, have much more troublesome post-ictal phenomena, including short-lived episodes of manic behaviour, depression of florid schizophrenia-like psychoses, confusional states, fugues and automatisms. These usually resolve within a few days and generally do not require additional medication provided the patient is in a safe environment with competent staff. They can be managed, if necessary, by transfer to the on-site Hospital Block in a residential epilepsy centre, with return to the classroom as soon as the child has recovered sufficiently.

Anti-epileptic drug problems: Adverse effects of medication such as sedation, dizziness, weight-gain or behavioural problems can often be managed on an outpatient basis by reducing or changing the medication. However, in cases where previous attempts to achieve this have been unsuccessful, or when it is difficult to distinguish subtle seizures from the adverse drug effects, residential management may be desirable. Because withdrawal seizures commonly occur when anti-epileptic drugs are reduced, it is highly desirable to carry out the drug changes under close medical supervision. If status epilepticus during the drug changeover is considered to be a risk, close supervision is mandatory. Depending on the anticipated length of the changeover, the child might be admitted to hospital for varying periods of time. Since the period required is often prolonged, the child would be liable to miss not only a significant amount of schooling, but also the opportunity to mix with a suitable peer group over that period. These difficulties are avoided by attendance at the residential epilepsy special school.

Inadequate medical control of seizures: Medical control of seizures may be deemed to be inadequate even if the seizures are not frequent. For example, even infrequent drop attacks or status epilepticus may be potentially serious enough to merit special residential schooling (Besag, 1988).

Difficult-to-recognise epilepsy: Although the term epilepsy makes most people think of the major seizure in which the sufferer falls to the ground and jerks violently, there are, however, many more subtle forms of seizures, notably the absence seizure and the complex partial seizure. Besag (1988) emphasisis that short-lived absence seizures can be a major handicap to learning and social interaction, but they may not be readily recognised. A child can have hundreds of absence seizures a day and these can interfere in a major way both with learning and social interaction. If the teachers do not recognise this condition, the child's apparent inattentiveness or withdrawal may be met with disciplinary measures. Complex partial seizures may lead to apparently bizarre behaviour which can sometimes be misinterpreted. Epigastric auras may be interpreted as nervousness rather than as a manifestation of epilepsy.

The accurate diagnosis of subtle seizures sometimes requires not only good observation but also the use of specialised EEG equipment. In addition to standard EEG machines, many residential epilepsy centres such as Lingfield Hospital School have facilities for twenty-four hour EEG monitoring, using a small portable device which monitors seizures by triggering a flashing lapel badge light whilst simultaneously logging the duration of the seizure on a digital display. A full assessment of children with these types of seizures in a residential setting may sometimes allow for a return to mainstream schooling after medication review and a full explanation of the situation to both the parents and the teaching staff.

Other Medical Problems

For those children who have additional medical problems such as major congenital heart disease, diabetes, hypopituitarism, hydrocephalus, chronic respiratory disease or epilepsy following accidents or neurosurgery, the twenty-four hour medical and nursing cover in a residential setting is of particular value. The presence of another major medical condition may add to the difficulty of educating the child in mainstream schooling. The team of psychologists, physiotherapists, occupational therapists and speech therapists together with the medical, nursing and teaching staff can combine in devising a total management plan to fulfil the special needs of each individual child.

Cognitive Problems

A large proportion of children with epilepsy referred to residential special schools have cognitive deficits (Besag, 1988). A careful assessment by the neuropsychologist, as part of the multi-disciplinary team, is essential if the child is to be managed appropriately and with understanding.

Behaviour Problems

According to Besag (1988), quite severe behaviour problems can develop in some children with epilepsy. Although drug treatment and the response of other people to the epilepsy (e.g. overprotection or rejection) can undoubtedly play a role, there may also be important neuropsychological factors responsible for the behaviour change. Some children have marked prodromes lasting hours or days before a seizure. During this time, they may become irritable, argumentative and even aggressive. The symptoms resolve when the seizure occurs.

Peer Group Problems

Besag (1988) states that the only child with epilepsy in a mainstream school may be subjected to unmerciful teasing. If they are also underachieving, their self-esteem may plummet and further withdrawal from the peer group may result. While, ideally, one might hope to help the child and the family to come to terms with the situation without removing the child from the school, this is not always plausible. Children with frequent subtle seizures may find group interactions of any kind very difficult and may also tend to withdraw. In a residential special school for epilepsy the condition is accepted, and its management is tailored according to the special needs. Peers who have similar problems readily accept the child.

Family and Social Problems

The degree of marital stress between parents of children with problematic epilepsy appears to be very high and the marriage break-up rate is accordingly very high (Besag, 1988). Sibling interactions may also become disturbed, other siblings either resenting the relative lack of attention they are shown or being ashamed of the person with epilepsy. One of the roles of the epilepsy centre or residential school is to bring families with similar problems together for mutual support and guidance from the professional team.

A significant number of children in epilepsy centres do not have parents who are able to look after them. Some have epilepsy because they have been subjected to non-accidental injury and have been taken into care. The families of other children may have separated for a variety of reasons directly or indirectly related to the epilepsy. For such children, the continuity of care in a residential special school may confer considerable benefits.

Psychiatric Problems

Interictal psychoses are relatively rare but can sometimes be florid and lead to considerable disturbance. Besag (1988) believes that if they occur against a setting of intellectual impairment much less upset may result if they can be managed in the setting of the residential school rather than transferring the child to the unfamiliar surroundings of a psychiatric hospital. However, in order to deal with these problems, psychiatric expertise must be readily available.

Brief post-ictal psychoses or affective disorders can also occur, usually taking the form of either paranoid ideation or of a depressive episode. If the symptoms are not severe, it is reasonable to wait for them to subside without giving additional medication, but this again necessitates the presence of staff who understand the nature of the problem and are competent in its management.

Other psychiatric problems can occur in children and adolescents with epilepsy, just as they can occur in the general population. Besag (1988) states that it would be just as foolish to attribute everything to the epilepsy as it would be to ignore the possible role of the epilepsy when managing these conditions. For these reasons, Besag (1988) argues that it is appropriate to deal with them within the setting of the residential school, drawing on outside consultants as necessary.

Multiple Problems

Any combination of the problems already listed can, of course, occur. Each individual problem might be adequately managed in the local setting, but the combination of them may create such difficulties that specialist residential schooling remains the only reasonable option.

The multiple problems can interact, exacerbating each other. In some cases, the residential school has a dramatic effect on children with such problems. They are introduced into an accepting peer group and provided with an individual programme designed by the multi-disciplinary team to make best use of their abilities and to boost self-esteem. Continuity of care is provided by all the staff on site and the children are encouraged to carry out activities which they might otherwise never had an opportunity to experience. In this environment, the problems sometimes rapidly resolve and interestingly, the seizure frequency may reduce.

Until 1981, there were six residential schools specialising in the treatment of children with epilepsy in England. However, the 1981 Education Act, which was enacted in 1983, aimed at integrating these special schools into mainstream education. This is in accordance with mainstream politics and is based on economic demands for more efficient methods of education (Aldenkamp et al., 1989). However, De Jong et al. (1997) argue that current attempts to adopt the Anglo-Saxon model of integration and 'educational mainstreaming' of children with epilepsy is inspired by economical instead of educational needs. Nevertheless, following the trend for the integration of those with epilepsy needs into mainstream education, the number of residential epilepsy schools has now been reduced to three.

The largest of these is St. Piers Lingfield Hospital School in Surrey, which has medium and long-term placements. The David Lewis Centre in Cheshire, accepts both children and adults for medium-term intensive assessments in a designated assessment centre. It also provides for long-term placements. St. Elizabeth's School in Much Hadham, Hertfordshire also offers long-term placements. While the Park Hospital for Children in Oxford has comprehensive facilities, it is generally used for relatively short and medium-term intensive inpatient assessments and reviews, the children remaining there for weeks or months rather than years.

In the special residential epilepsy schools the emphasis is on allowing the child to take full part in educational and social activities. A strong emphasis is placed on relationships with the community, both locally and further afield. Although this does not differ, in principle, from what should happen in any other school, it is possible to offer a broader curriculum and a much wider range of activities to children with severe or problematic epilepsy because of the training and experience of the staff. De Jong et al. (1997) takes the view that there is a lack of knowledge among teachers in regular school settings concerning epilepsy specific variables (e.g. side effects of AEDs) in the aetiology of educational problems.

Another important advantage of the residential centres is the opportunities which such centres provide for anti-epileptic drug reviews. Besag (1987) notes that the concept of admitting a child with epilepsy to hospital for two or three weeks often has little basis in reality. A common situation is that the child is admitted to hospital and, because of the changed environment, the seizures improve. When the child is later discharged the seizures recommence. The residential centre, in contrast, has the opportunity of observing the child in a number of situations over a period of weeks before instituting any changes. In general, assessment of anti-epileptic drug changes cannot be hurried. Although some children will respond immediately to a drug change, others may take several weeks to respond. In contrast to the hospital settings, the residential centres offer education, recreation, leisure, a peer group and much opportunity for interaction with the world outside.

The residential special school can also fulfill a role in the pre-surgical assessment and the post-surgical rehabilitation of children undergoing epilepsy neurosurgery. Abolition of seizures may imply a major change in life-role and some children and teenagers find it very difficult to come to terms with this and may require much support.

As well as providing education and care for children with epilepsy, Besag (1987) believes that these residential schools play an important role as a research and resource facility. Research on new anti-epileptic medication can be conducted much more safely when the children are being observed 24 hours a day in an establishment which has an on-site doctor, with full EEG and nursing facilities. The epilepsy centres have provided the basis for important research into drug treatment, cognitive changes and behavioural disturbance in children with epilepsy over the years.

A further important role of the residential schools is to provide teaching and training for other professionals. Information is provided and understanding promoted through conferences, seminars and parent meetings. The recent trend in the UK has been for the centres to join with the epilepsy associations in holding courses for teachers, general practitioners, doctors and other staff who have responsibility for the management of children with epilepsy outside the centres. Morrow (1993) takes issue with Besag's cases for the retention of special residential centres for children with epilepsy. He contends that the practice of removing patients with epilepsy from the realm of general physicians and general neurologists may result in a gradual erosion of the skills of these professionals because it lessens their exposure to epilepsy. Protagonists of specialised centres would argue, however, that increasing the specialisation in epilepsy in these centres should increase knowledge and expertise and improve the management of epilepsy in general. The setting of the specialised clinic would allow other members of a multi-disciplinary team to attend. It would be unlikely that there would be any erosion in the skills of other physicians involved in the care of epilepsy, as the number of patients with epilepsy is so large that there would be little problem with the general services co-existing with the specialised clinics.

6.4   EDUCATIONAL LEGISLATION IN ENGLAND

Until the 19th century, the main source of assistance for persons with epilepsy was to be found in the lunatic asylums. Grant (1981) recounts that by the mid 1800s segregated provision had appeared, with the consequent establishment of epileptic colonies (institutions where persons with epilepsy were confined). Concern with education of children with epilepsy was a relatively recent innovation and until the end of the 19th century most children with epilepsy received no education at all (Kurtz, 1983). In the early days of formal education little provision was made for children with a handicap and they struggled to cope in large classes where the curriculum was geared to the 'normal' child (Rogan, 1980).

In 1896, the British Education Department established a 'Committee on Defective and Epileptic Children' which proposed that children who experienced seizures less frequently than once a month could attend ordinary classes. However, it recommended that local education authorities should provide special residential schools or, alternatively, pay for children who were subject to more than one epileptic seizure a month to be educated in voluntary institutions. It was also recommended that, by law, all children with epilepsy should be required to attend school. Due to what was considered excessive costs and a too heavy organisational demand on the School Boards, many of these recommendations were shelved (Rogan, 1980).

In 1899, the Elementary Education (Defective and Epileptic Children) Act merely allowed school boards to provide special education for mentally and physically defective and epileptic children. Ten years after the passing of the Act only 40% (n=133) of local authorities had taken advantage of the enhanced rate of grant available to them to make the special provision for handicapped children. It was not until the passing of the Education Act in 1918 (when the powers given in the 1899 legislation were converted into a duty) that compulsory provision of education for the child with epilepsy became a reality (DES, 1978). However, by the time the Act was passed in 1918 there were already six residential schools specifically designated for the education of the child with epilepsy.

The 1921 Education Act laid down the general framework for special education provision. It treated the education of handicapped children as an entirely separate category of provision, stating that handicapped pupils could only be educated in special schools or special classes. 'Epileptic' continued to be a recognised category of handicap, along with the blind, deaf and defective. It was the parents' responsibility to ensure that their child attended an appropriate school, from seven to 16 years of age (Cull and Brown, 1989). Even so, children with epilepsy continued to be disadvantaged, as exemplified by a survey in Surrey in 1928. This survey reported that, of the children with epilepsy of school-age, 20% were attending residential schools for epilepsy but 25% of educable children were not attending any school (Tylor Fox, 1928).

Following the publication of the Board of Education Green Paper- 'Education after the War' in 1941, and the subsequent White Paper, 'Education Reconstruction', a new Education Bill was presented to parliament. Parliamentary debate brought to the fore the sentiment that it was time for a single framework of education to be established in which special education would have a natural place. The 1944 Education Act paved the way towards integrated education for less seriously handicapped children and placed upon the Minister of Education the duty of making regulations which would define the different groups of children for which special provision should be made. Those with serious disabilities, of which epilepsy was considered to be one, continued to be educated in either day or residential special schools. Attendance at school was now required between five and 16 years, with the right to remain beyond 16 years of age. These regulations were produced in 1945 and ruled that children with epilepsy were seriously disabled and must be educated in special residential or day schools (Rogan, 1980).

In England during the 1950s, two reports concerning people with epilepsy were published. The first, published by the Ministry of Health 1953, was concerned with their special welfare needs. Amongst many recommendations it was advised that separate accommodation should be provided in the epileptic colonies (or 'centres' as they were then labelled), for (a) the 'low grade', (b) the 'difficult' and (c) those requiring short-term stabilisation. Of more importance was the subsequent Report of the Cohen Committee (Ministry of Health, 1956). It recommended that the epileptic centres should be as much therapeutic as custodial, and that they should be concerned not only with the medical care but also with the rehabilitation of patients, ultimately returning them to a normal life in the community (Grant, 1981).

However, it was not until the Reid Report (Department of Health and Social Security and Welsh Office, 1969) that progress began to take place. Of a total of 56 recommendations, 12 concerned the epileptic colonies and the proposed new concept of special centres. The Reid Report provided the basis on which the present special centres in England are based (Grant, 1981). It was stressed that, with good co-ordination between family doctors and the hospital and local authority services, the vast majority of people with epilepsy could be given a high standard of care in the community, based on a multi-disciplinary approach and including an extension of special epilepsy clinics. It was recommended that the latter should be at district general hospital level as well as in regional neurosurgical centres, and that they should form part of appropriate hospital departments such as neurology, psychiatry or paediatrics. Nevertheless, it was recognised that a small but significant number of people with epilepsy required even more specialised attention because of continued seizures, and that there were also those who required medical supervision under ordinary living and working conditions. The concept of 'special centres' was introduced and it was recommended that these should comprise of the following:

1. A hospital neurological and neurosurgical unit containing all the necessary facilities for diagnosis and treatment.
2. A residential unit to which appropriate people with epilepsy could be admitted for a period of care, after an established diagnosis and assessment has been made.

Although the "ineducable" status category was abolished in 1970, it was not until 1976 that the Education Act required that all handicapped children, including those with epilepsy, should be educated in mainstream schools, wherever possible (DES, 1978).

In 1978, a Committee under the chairmanship of Baroness Warnock was established to look into special education in England and Wales and to present its findings to the Secretary of State. In relation to children with epilepsy, the Warnock Report (Committee of Enquiry into Education of Handicapped Children and Young People, HMSO, 1978) recommended that in order to create the right attitudes to children with epilepsy, every effort should be made to inform staff in schools and colleges about the facts of epilepsy, how it may be controlled by drugs, the side effects of drugs and how it should be managed, should seizures occur. The Report advised that lack of full knowledge might cause a child's activities to be unduly restricted, and if the school did not know about the existence of the condition the child may run unnecessary risks. It was noted that even where satisfactory control of seizures by anti-convulsants was achieved, many children with epilepsy had serious concentration and behaviour problems which affected their learning, and better arrangements for reviewing their progress were advised.

The Warnock Report (1978) noted that some children with epilepsy needed to go to residential special schools, either because their seizures were difficult to control or because they had additional or associated disabilities or difficulties which made unreasonable demands on ordinary schools and their families. It was recommended that the function of the six residential special schools for children with epilepsy be reconsidered and that there should be at least one residential special school in each region where expertise in the multi-professional assessment and approach to the health, care and education of children with epilepsy was developed.

The 1981 Education Act, which was enacted in 1983, further enhanced and supported the opportunities for integrated education. Within the context of this Act, children were no longer seen as falling into a particular category of handicap, but rather as having Special Educational Needs. In this way the Act attempted to take into account the whole child as an individual, including his strengths as well as his weaknesses, rather than just concentrating on his disability. Once a child was identified as having Special Educational Needs, a formal document or written statement of those needs, presented in a prescribed format, was required. This statement had to incorporate educational, medical and psychological advice and specify the type of educational provision considered most appropriate, the type of school, and additional non-educational provision where relevant. Parents were to be advised when such an assessment was being made and they could make their own contribution to the statement, in addition to which they had a right of appeal (Statutory Instruments (1983) The Education, (Special Educational Needs) Regulations 1983. HMSO: London).

It was not envisaged that procedures for making enforceable statements of special needs provision would be required for most children with epilepsy. As Circular 1/83 (paragraph 15) states, ".. formal procedures would not be required where ordinary schools provide special educational provision from their own resources in the form of additional tuition and remedial provision, or in normal circumstances, where the child attends a reading centre or unit for disruptive pupils." It was considered that these provisions should be adequate for most children with epilepsy who have statements of special needs. The key factor in deciding whether to seek a statement of special needs would most probably be in those cases where extra resources, in terms of staffing or equipment, would be required to cater for such needs in the ordinary school (Circular 8/81, paragraph 9). In these cases, it was intimated that the Secretary of State expected Local Education Authorities to afford the protection of a statement to all children who had severe or complex learning difficulties which required the provision of extra resources in ordinary schools (Circular 1/83, paragraph 14). This encompassed the child with epilepsy who had additional problems. However, it was recognised that from time to time a child with epilepsy may also require the protection of an official statement within the ordinary school setting.

The 1981 Education Act also noted that there would continue to remain a need, including that for residential provision, for some children with multiple handicaps, including epilepsy, to be placed in special schools. The decision would be based on an individual assessment. For all children with epilepsy who have statements, reassessment was to be mandatory when the child was thirteen and a half years old, if the last assessment was performed before the child was twelve and a half.

The 1981 Education Act also referred to provision for children below school age and those remaining after the age of 16. Both of these provisions are particularly relevant to children with epilepsy, since research had confirmed the benefits of early intervention and also, in some cases, of extended schooling to compensate for developmental or educational delays. In order to assist in the identification of younger children with special educational needs, Section 10 of the Act placed an obligation on Health Authorities to inform parents of these provisions for children under the age of five so that the benefits of early assessment and intervention could be realised.

The 1993 Education Act introduced the Code of Practice on the identification and assessment of pupils with special educational needs. The Code laid down the key principles and procedures, based on accepted good practice, for the systematic identification and assessment of special educational needs. Under Section 166 of the Education Act (1993) a Health Authority must provide help to a Local Education Authority for a pupil with special educational needs, unless the Health Authority considers that the help is not necessary to enable the LEA to carry out its duties. This applies whether or not the pupil attends a special school. Help from the Health Authority could include providing advice and training for school staff in procedures dealing with a child's medical needs if that child would otherwise have limited access to education. It recommended that health and educational authorities and schools should work together in close partnership with parents to ensure proper support in school for pupils with medical needs.

The 1993 Education Act was repealed in November 1996 and the law on special education is now contained in the 1996 Education Act. This was a consolidating Act and there were no changes of substance to the law on special education (Came and Webster, 1999). Special educational needs (SEN) in the United Kingdom are seen as undergoing the most far-reaching review for 20 years. A comprehensive agenda for SEN, outlined in two Green Papers for England and Wales, has been initiated through the 'Programme of Action'. The current government's Programme of Action (October 1998) announced its intention to produce a revised Code that will come into effect during the school year 2000/2001.

6.5 EDUCATIONAL PROVISION FOR CHILDREN WITH EPILEPSY IN THE REPUBLIC OF IRELAND

6.5.1 Introduction

About one person in every two hundred or nearly 20,000 people in Ireland have some form of epilepsy (Brainwave, 1991). As a large proportion of people have their first seizure before the age of twenty, many children of schoolgoing age are affected by the condition. Research conducted by Thompson (1987) in England indicates that children with epilepsy are at a significant risk of developing learning difficulties, with problems occuring in between five and 50 per cent of such children. For the student with epilepsy multiple factors influence his or her abilities and school performance. These varying educational and emotional difficulties experienced by many children with epilepsy are outlined in Chapter 5.

In the following section, the development of special education in Ireland is briefly examined and the existence of educational provision for students with epilepsy in the Republic of Ireland is reviewed. Education acts and reports are examined in order to establish the legislative implications regarding provision for children with epilepsy. It should be noted in this context that research in this area proved to be very difficult and was not facilitated by any of the agencies of State entrusted with either the care or the education of children with special needs. Despite numerous telephone calls and letters to the Department of Health and the Special Education Section in the Department of Education and Science (Appendix 3/9), the researcher was unable to obtain any official declaration of policy on the kinds of special educational provision that are made available to children with epilepsy. A letter to the Minister for Education and Science, Micheal Martin T.D., was finally acknowledged in June, 1999 (Appendix 3) and enquiries were reported to be underway, but no response has since been received.

6.5.2 An Overview of Special Educational Provision in the Republic of Ireland

The nineteenth century marked the growth of special education in Ireland. It was greatly influenced by religious orders and voluntary non-statutory bodies, private donations and the efforts of parents. The State played little role in this growth, although at times they did support the initiatives of these groups (Department of Education, 1983). As was the case in many countries, special educational services were initially provided for those who had visual, auditory and physical impairments (McDonnell, 1992). Following this provision, the Poor Relief (Ireland) Acts of 1838 and 1847 and the Poor Afflicted Persons (Relief) Act of 1878 were introduced to provide services for mentally handicapped persons. Such services included residential care in psychiatric hospitals, county homes and hospitals for the physically disabled (Department of Education and Health 1983). However, the educational needs of children with mental handicap were neglected until the middle of the twentieth century as they were considered to be ineducable (Department of Education and Health, 1993). Individuals with epilepsy were included in this group.

Expansion in special schooling, especially for children with mental handicap, did not take place until the mid-1950s (McGee, 1990). The provision of services for the mentally handicapped in Ireland was first examined through a Commission of Inquiry into the Reformatory and Industrial School System (1936) and later by a Commission of Inquiry on Mental Handicap (1965). According to Coolahan (1981), the latter Report "..reflected a new awareness of the problems of educating the mentally handicapped and a greater social concern generally that the problems should be grappled with." The Report of the Commission of Inquiry on Mental Handicap (1965) made many recommendations which influenced the development of educational provision for the mentally handicapped, and following its publication, there was a considerable increase in the establishment of special schools. This report also recognised that mentally handicapped pupils would benefit from a curriculum which could be adjusted to suit their needs. Such a curriculum was made available through the Department of Education in 1971 and most special schools and special classes in mainstream schools provided a modified curriculum for their pupils. The Report of the Commission of Inquiry on Mental Handicap (1965) adopted the use of the term 'mental handicap' and "of the three levels, mild, moderate and severe, insofar as an intelligence quotient can be regarded as a measure of mental handicap." Arising from this report, there was a slow expansion of special schools and classes in mainstream schools, as well as both day and residential provision.

During the 1970s there was a shift from segregation in special schools to integration into mainstream schools for children with special educational needs. This shift was influenced by the British 1970 (Handicapped) Act which required that all mentally retarded children should be provided with appropriate educational placement. The issue of integration for all handicapped persons was officially addressed by the White Paper on Educational Development (1980). However, the support services required for successful integration were not fully in place in ordinary schools (Department of Education, 1980) and the pace of integration has been slow.

The Report of the Primary Education Review Body (1990) indicated that significant developments had occurred in primary education in the area of integration of children with handicaps since the Commission on Inquiry on Mental Handicap in 1965. Some of these developments included:
1. The implementation of the new curriculum for primary schools in 1971.
2. The pursuit of a policy of integration for children with handicaps by the Department of Education.

3. A major review of services for the mentally handicapped by the Department of Health. This review postulates that mild mental handicap should be considered as part of the general problem of learning disability rather than be included in the field of mental handicap (Department of Education, 1990).

Following a recommendation of the Report of the Primary Education Review Body (1990) the Special Education Review Committee was established in 1991 with terms of reference which can be summarised as follows:
To report and make recommendations on the educational provision for children with special needs with regard to-
(1) Identification and assessment processes
(2) Appropriate educational provision
(3) Support services
(4) Linkages between the Department of Education and other Departments and Services

The Report of the Special Education Review Committee (1993) indicated that separate educational provision had evolved for children in the following categories of handicap:
(a) Mild mental handicap
(b) Moderate mental handicap
(c) Severe and profound mental handicap
(d) Emotional disturbance
(e) Physical handicap
(f) Visual impairment
(g) Hearing impairment
(h) Language disorders and specific reading disabilities
        (Department of Education, 1994)

The Report of the Special Education Review Committee (SERC, 1993) defined students with special needs as including *".. all those whose disabilities and/or circumstances prevent or hinder them from benefiting adequately from the education which is normally provided for pupils of the same age, or for whom the education which can generally be provided in the ordinary classroom is not sufficiently challenging."*

Although a detailed submission was made by Brainwave, the Irish Epilepsy Association to the Special Education Review Committee (1993), its recommendations were not included in the final report. In fact, no reference whatsoever was made to the position of children with epilepsy within the Irish school system. Among the recommendations submitted by Brainwave, the Irish Epilepsy Association was the need for the establishment of an assessment service specifically catering for children with epilepsy where appropriate medical, psychological and educational programmes could be designed to meet individual children's needs. This assessment service would consist of a multidisciplinary team with expertise in educational and neuropsychological assessment. Such an assessment could take a number of weeks or longer and would require residential facilities for EEG monitoring, drug manipulations, behaviour therapy and work with the family.   In England and Wales, there are four such specialist assessment units and educational facilities (Thompson 1987; Cull and Brown, 1989).

The need for a special education facility for children with severe epilepsy and associated problems was also recommended in the submission to the Review Committee on Special Education (1993). Besag (1987) believes that children with difficult epilepsy need specialised multi-disciplinary services, depending on the severity of their problems and that the special school catering for children with other handicaps is not always in a position to meet the educational and medical needs of these children. Although current thinking subscribes to the theory of integrated education, Brainwave, the Irish Epilepsy Association (1991) states that there is still a role for a special educational facility for children who have complicated epilepsy and severe learning difficulties interacting with other neurological, environmental and psychological problems. However, Brainwave considers that this need could also be assessed by the establishment of a multidisciplinary assessment unit which would evaluate the possibility of continuing mainstream or special education for children with epilepsy and would prevent inappropriate referrals to special education, as happens under the current practice.

In response to the SERC Report, a conference was held at the Belfield campus of University College Dublin 1994. While Brainwave made no written submission to the conference, the conference proceedings also made no specific mention of the special educational needs of children with epilepsy (Spelman and Griffin, 1994).

The Report on the Status of People with Disabilities (1996) found that approximately 4% of the school-going population have disabilities and special educational needs in Ireland. Special schools cater for about 8,000 of these but there are approximately 3,800 students with a variety of disabilities in special classes in mainstream primary schools. A further 8,000 students with 'specific disabilities' are in mainstream classes in primary schools. At second level, approximately 2,300 students with disabilities are catered for in special classes but there are no statistics available for those who are not in a special class.

In contrast with the rest of Europe, there has been relatively little legislation governing education in Ireland until the Education Act (1998). The purpose of the Education Act (1998) with reference to the education of pupils with special educational needs, is as follows:
> "*An Act to make provision in the interests of the common good for the education of every person in the state, including any person with a disability or who has other special educational needs.*"

However, no specific reference is made in the Act to the position of children with epilepsy and their educational needs.

The National Council for Curriculum and Assessment (NCCA) was established by the Minister of Education in November 1987 to conduct a continuing review of matters relating to curriculum and assessment procedures for primary and second level education. The Education Act (1998) sets out the legislation to establish the NCCA as a statutory body. The Act specifically states that a function of the Council of the NCCA shall be ".. to advise the Minister on the requirements, as regards curriculum and syllabuses, of students with a disability or other special educational needs" [S41.2 (f)] The work of the NCCA in relation to Special Education has taken into account the findings of the SERC Report (1993). Epilepsy was not included or defined by the SERC Report (1993) as an area of special educational need. As the work of the NCCA, in relation to special education, takes into account the findings of the SERC Report (1993) its current deliberations make no reference to the educational needs of children with epilepsy.

The only existing official provision made by the Irish Department of Education and Science for students with epilepsy would appear to be in the area of state examinations. Special arrangements exist for candidates with epilepsy who are sitting state examinations. These include:
(1) The provision of a separate room and supervisor if requested by the principal of the school.
(2) If a student has a seizure during an examination he or she will not be given extra time to finish the paper but will be marked on the part of the paper which has been completed as if it were the full examination. However, in order to qualify for this special consideration candidates must have applied in November of the previous year.

Brainwave, the Irish Epilepsy Association (1991) feel that these arrangements do not cover the full range of difficulties faced by a student with epilepsy. If a person has a seizure before an examination and misses a full paper there is no facility to repeat. Brainwave (1998) also comments that not all schools are aware of such considerations and therefore do not apply for them. Students who have partial or 'petit mal' seizures may be refused because of the difficulty of proving their occurrence.

Inquiries to the Department of Education and Science regarding their policy on the availability of the Home Tuition Scheme for students with epilepsy who have missed a lot of school were also unanswered (Appendix 3). However, the researcher is aware of one student who, following long negotitions between the Department of Education and Science and his neurologist, secured one hour's home tuition per week.

6.6   SUMMARY
This chapter provided an overview of the development of special educational provision in both

Ireland and England, with particular reference to legislation which catered for the needs of pupils with epilepsy.

Most children with epilepsy will have their seizures largely controlled and will attend mainstream education. This is in accordance with current thinking which subscribes to the theory of integrated education. Brainwave, the Irish Epilepsy Association supports the view that integration is acceptable as an overall policy, and believes that it should not be seen as necessary to have separate educational facilities for children with epilepsy. Instead the child or young person is best served by having the company of peers who can grow to understand the condition and in turn assist in the development of self-esteem and enhanced performance.

Although Brainwave seeks to encourage the education of children with epilepsy in mainstream schools, it also recognises the need for special schooling for a sub-population of children who have a drug-resistant or severe form of epilepsy. A review of provision for children with special educational needs showed that children with severe epilepsy and its associated problems are not catered for in the Irish educational system. Ireland is the only country in the EU that has no special educational or assessment facilities for children with more difficult forms of epilepsy (Brainwave, the Irish Epilepsy Association, 1991). The Irish Epilepsy Association is aware of a number of children being sent to residential schools in Britain due to lack of facilities in Ireland. However, inquiries to the Department of Education and Science regarding the number of such children were not answered (Appendix 3). In a meeting with Dr. Frank Besag, medical director of Lingfield Hospital School, Surrey, the researcher was told how an Irish pupil had just completed his schooling there in June 1999. In view of this, it would appear that sufficient provision for children with special educational needs, as a result of their epilepsy, is not being made by the State in recognition of their constitutional right to education.

Among the fundamental rights ascribed to the citizens of the Republic of Ireland in the Constitution of 1937, is the right of children to 'receive an education appropriate to their abilities, aptitudes and potential.' Almost sixty years later, the recognition of this right was reiterated in the White Paper on Education (1995). In order that the educational needs of all children be met, certain provisions for those with special needs are essential. O'Toole (1998) believes that it is a truism to state that the best test of a democracy is the manner in which it treats its minorities. He believes that if we were to apply this test to the Irish education system at present, it would come out very badly indeed. Certainly in the area of provision for children with epilepsy, this would appear to be the case. Placement in a special school for children with mental, physical or emotional handicap, as is the current practice, is not the type of educational provision children with epilepsy either benefit from or deserve.

In summary therefore, the 1990s have seen the publication of six major educational policy documents in Ireland, the most recent of which is the most far-reaching Education Act since the foundation of the State. In none of these documents is any reference whatsoever made to the special educational needs of children with epilepsy. Further, these children do not even come under the definitions of children with special needs as cited in any of these documents. Therefore, it may legitimately be concluded that children with epilepsy do not have any entitlement to any specific form of special educational provision, whether integrated or otherwise, nor does any such entitlement exist in law within the Republic of Ireland. This situation appears to stand in stark contradiction to the legislative injunction which the Irish Education Act (1998) places on the school system: '.. that recognised schools shall provide education to students which is appropriate to their abilities and needs….and ensure that the educational needs of all students, including those with a disability or other special educational needs are identified and provided for' [S9 (a)].

In the broader context of child welfare, equality and disability legislation, there is no doubt that the last decade has witnessed a heightened awareness of the rights of children with special educational needs in the Republic of Ireland, and some quite significant developments in special needs education have occurred. These developments are comprehensively reviewed within the context of provision for people with epilepsy in Chapter 10.

CHAPTER SEVEN

THE RESEARCH DESIGN: NATURE AND PURPOSE OF THE ENQUIRY

7.1 OVERVIEW OF THE EMPIRICAL ENQUIRY

The number of children with epilepsy of school-going age in the Republic of Ireland warrants urgent and appropriate medical and educational intervention and is of major concern to parents. Over recent years, in both Europe and the United States, a number of reputable studies have researched the problems of children with epilepsy (Rutter et al., 1970; Sillanpaa 1973, Ross et al., 1980, Ellenberg et al., 1985). While no Irish statistics are available on the incidence/prevalence of epilepsy, comparative U.S. and U.K. studies would indicate that at least one in every 200, or 20,000 people in Ireland could be affected by epilepsy (Brainwave, the Irish Epilepsy Association, 1998).

To date, no research whatsoever on the incidence of epilepsy among schoolgoing children has been carried out in the Republic of Ireland. Indeed, it appears that, at present there is no co-ordinated body of information available in any Governmental Department or Health Board concerning such basic and essential information as the number of children and adults with epilepsy in the State. Nor are children with epilepsy (the diagnosis of which is often uncertain) recognised for any category of special education provision by the State Department of Education and Science.

The empirical aspects of this study seek to determine the experiences of parents of children with epilepsy and their views on the provision currently made available to them in the Republic of Ireland. A sample of parents whose children have epilepsy were surveyed through a detailed postal questionnaire in order to ascertain their experiences of and views concerning the medical and educational provision and general service delivery afforded their children. The results of this investigation are outlined and discussed in Chapter 8.

The present study reviewed the research from the United Kingdom, the United States and Europe in an effort to establish its relevance to children with epilepsy in Ireland. Chapter 1 considers the nature of epilepsy. The various meanings of the word epilepsy are examined and classifications and types of seizures are identified. The aetiology, triggers and epidemiology of epilepsy are also considered.

Chapter 2 examines historical conceptions of epilepsy. It identifies the various historical terms which were given to the condition, and examines how those labels demonstrated people's beliefs about the condition. Relevant developments in the medical field of research in the 19th and 20th centuries are briefly summarised, and the various laws relating to epilepsy are reviewed.

Chapter 3 examines attitudes towards and beliefs about epilepsy from an historical perspective, and considers their implications for the ways in which epilepsy is viewed today. The issue of stigma, as it applies to epilepsy, and the factors that contribute to these attitudes are considered.

Chapter 4 considers the family's adjustment to the condition. It examines the reactions evoked by the diagnosis and the ensuing impact on family life. Restrictions imposed, both on the child and the family are analysed, and parental concerns relating to medical, educational and future aspects of the child's welfare are identified.

Chapter 5 reviews the findings of a number of major international studies on educational attainment and learning difficulties among children with epilepsy. The causes of learning disabilities and behavioural disturbance, as related to epilepsy, are also explored.

Chapter 6 documents the educational provision for children with epilepsy, both in Ireland and England. It looks at the historical development of the epilepsy centres in England and other countries, and their present-day role in the provision for people with epilepsy. The reasons for referral to schools for children with epilepsy are also examined. Educational legislation in England and Wales is also briefly outlined. In the final section, educational legislation and provision for children with epilepsy in the Republic of Ireland is considered.

Chapter 8 provides an analysis of the survey findings relating to the parents' experiences of and views concerning the medical and educational provision and general service delivery currently made available to their children in the Republic of Ireland.

Chapter 9 reviews the results of the empirical study in light of relevant research findings elsewhere. Educational and medical implications arising from the findings are analysed, and recommendations with specific relevance for the Departments of Health and Education and Science are made. The chapter concludes with a summary statement of the 21 recommendations of greatest significance for the future medical and educational care of children with epilepsy in Ireland.

Chapter 10 puts the findings of the study in perspective by reviewing them within the context of an interview conducted with the Chief Executive of Brainwave, the Irish Epilepsy Association. The findings and recommendations are also examined within the context of the present Irish legislative and constitutional environment.

7.2   AIMS OF THE STUDY
The overall aim of the empirical aspect of this study was to survey the parents of children defined as having epilepsy in order to obtain a comprehensive view of the medical and educational provision afforded them in Ireland. The aims of the study may be summarised as follows:
To compile information on the biographical details and family circumstances of the children in the survey.
- To collate information on family history of epilepsy and birth circumstances of the children.
- To record the developmental history of the children.
- To compile information on the nature and effectiveness of the children's initial medical referral, diagnosis and intervention.
- To obtain essential information regarding the types of drug-related regimes prescribed for the children, the parents' views as to their suitability and side-effects induced.
- To establish the effectiveness of the follow-up advisory and support services made available to the parents.
- To compile information on the kinds of educational provision to which children with epilepsy have access, and the extent to which such provision has met their special educational needs.
- To compile information on the educational experiences of the children and to note the general level of awareness within the school system of the particular nature and characteristics of children with epilepsy, and the extent to which the system is willing to provide appropriate forms of education for children with such characteristics.
- To obtain information on the social adjustment of children with epilepsy and the extent to which epilepsy has affected their relationships and social development.
- To note parents' concerns and expectations for their children's future and to compile their opinions of the Irish Educational System and the extent to which it has served their children's educational needs.
- To review the results of the empirical study in light of relevant research findings and to analyse the arising educational and medical implications.
- To compile a summary statement of the recommendations of greatest significance for the future medical and educational care of children with epilepsy.
- To provide an overview of provision for people with epilepsy within the context of the views expressed by the Chief Executive of Brainwave, the Irish Epilepsy Association, and also within the context of the present Irish legislative and constitutional environment.

7.3   CHOICE OF RESEARCH DESIGN
This study employs the survey approach, which may be described as descriptive research which is quantitative in nature. In order to collect data, postal questionnaires were devised and used as the primary data collection method.

According to Bell (1993), the aim of a questionnaire is to obtain information which can be anlaysed and patterns extracted and comparisons made. As described by Bailey (1994) and Frankfort and Nachmias (1996), there are certain advantages to adopting this method of research. In the case of this particular research, the questionnaire provided the most convenient access to a geographically dispersed sample at a relatively low cost. The questionnaire also provided a degree of anonymity for respondents. This is especially important when sensitive issues such as epilepsy are being studied.

However, the questionnaire method has certain limitations. For example, with no interviewer present, there can be no probing if the respondent's answer is too vague, or if the question asked is misunderstood. The response rate to a questionnaire can be low, as low as 10%, according to Bailey (1994). However, for the purpose of this study, the questionnaire method was considered the most suitable. In addition to baseline statistical data, the use of open-ended questions yielded valuable opinions and information. Such responses were subjected to a content analysis, which enabled individual responses to certain questions to be reported. The value of reporting individual interpretations to certain items on the questionnaire lies in the fact that it allows for respondents' views and opinions on an existing situation to be voiced. The questionnaire employed in the present study is described in full in Section 7.6.

7.4   DEVELOPMENT OF THE STUDY

Due to the lack of basic research data concerning children with epilepsy in the Republic of Ireland, there were no previous studies which could be consulted. Therefore, it was necessary to conduct substantial preparatory background work in order to obtain information about epilepsy, its medical determinations and current educational provision in Ireland. Throughout June and July 1998, preliminary contact was made with staff, agencies and associations involved in the service provision for children with epilepsy.

In preparation for the study, preliminary meetings were held in July and August 1998 with the Information Officer and Counsellor in Brainwave, the Irish Epilepsy Association, to discuss the most pertinent issues for parents of children with epilepsy.

The researcher also met with a small number of parents of children with epilepsy to gain insight into the difficulties encountered by their children with the existing medical and educational system.

As part of the preparation for the enquiry, an Epilepsy Awareness Day, organised by Brainwave, the Irish Epilepsy Association, and presented by recognised experts in the field of epilepsy, was attended in Dublin in September 1998.

Following conversations and correspondence with professionals in the Department of Health and the Department of Education and Science, it became evident that there was no database of school-going children with epilepsy from which a random number of parents could be surveyed. Therefore, it was necessary to have further meetings with personnel in Brainwave to discuss the possibility of using their members' list as a means of obtaining a sample of parents.

While researching educational legislation and provision in the Republic of Ireland, the researcher also interviewed Dr. Patricia Noonan Walshe, at the Centre for Developmental Disabilities, University College Dublin.

As part of the research into educational provision in England, the researcher met with Dr. Frank Besag, medical director of the renowned St. Piers Lingfield Hospital School in Surrey, England. By visiting the school and speaking with Dr. Besag, valuable insight into educational provision for children with epilepsy was gained.

7.5   SAMPLE

Following discussions with Brainwave, it was agreed that the sample of parents would be selected from the organisation's members' list. As their mailing list was not classified by category, this proved to be a difficult and time-consuming task. The objective was to determine which members were parents of school-going children with epilepsy. The sample was generated with the assistance of the Community Resource Officers in the regional branches across the country, as these Officers were most familiar with the names and circumstances of parents of school-going children with epilepsy in their regions. A total of 139 parents, who were geographically dispersed across the country, constituted the final sample.

7.6   INSTRUMENTATION
7.6.1 Parent Questionnaire
The research evidence reviewed in Chapters 1 to 6 suggested suitable questions and issues which should be included in the questionnaire (Appendix 4). The questionnaire, which was devised by the researcher under academic supervision, contained eight sections with 113 items in total. Care was taken to ensure that the items were as brief as possible, explicit and unambiguous. The questionnaire sought parents' opinions on and experiences of the following issues:

1. **Background Characteristics:** This included biographical details about the child, such as age, gender, family circumstances, including marital situation, number of children in the family, levels of education completed by the parents and their occupations. Family history of epilepsy, birth and pregnancy circumstances and the developmental history of the child were also represented in this section.

2. **Initial Referral and Diagnosis:** This included details about the particular behaviours that led the parents to suspect that something was wrong with their child and the age at which this occurred. Parents were also asked to report on referral procedures to specialists and the manner in which they were told about their child's condition. Information about types of counselling recommended and attended was requested. Reactions evoked by the diagnosis and the people they told about their child's condition were also included in this section.

3. **Medical Issues:** This included details about prescription and administration of drugs and their related side effects.

4. **Follow-Up Advisory and Support Services:** Details regarding reassessment, satisfaction with their child's monitoring and areas in which advice on management were given were surveyed in this section.

5. **Educational Provision:** This included information about the child's level and type of schooling. Parents were asked to report on their experiences when discussing their child's condition with the principal and teacher(s) in their child's school. Teachers' knowledge of and attitude to epilepsy was also surveyed, as were teachers' procedures following a seizure.

6. **Educational Attainment:** This section examined parental opinions about their child's progress at school, and the extent to which it was affected by their condition and prescribed medication. It included details about work missed and absenteeism due to their condition as well as the need for extra educational assistance. Parental awareness of Department of Education and Science subject and examination exemptions was also investigated.

7. **Social Adjustment:** The extent to which the children's condition affected their relationship with their siblings and friends was examined, as was their behaviour in school and at home. This section also included questions regarding the child's interests and participation in activities, parental restrictions and over-protection. Information about the child's self-confidence and general adjustment was also sought.

8. **The Future:** Parents' educational expectations for their child, their concerns regarding the future and their opinion about the type of school which would best provide for their child's specific needs were sought. Their views on how the school system has, or has not met the needs of their child as a pupil with epilepsy, in the Irish Educational System were requested in this final section of the questionnaire.

The questionnaire included a variety of response formats, including those which required yes/no answers or "tick the box". Other questions were open-ended and allowed the respondent to elaborate about personal experiences. Multiple choice and rank order questions were also employed.

7.6.2 Piloting the Questionnaire

According to Bailey (1994), piloting the questionnaire is the final stage in questionnaire construction and one of the most important. By administering a small number of questionnaires, flaws can be identified and rectified. Similarly, Bell (1993) advocates that all data gathering instruments should be piloted in order to test how long it takes the recipients to complete them, to check that all questions and instructions are clear, and to enable the researcher to remove any redundant questions.

Much of the initial drafting and piloting was conducted under academic supervision and with the assistance of fellow research students. The questionnaire was then posted to the Chief Executive of Brainwave, the Irish Epilepsy Association, on Friday 26th February 1999 for official piloting. A meeting was held two weeks later to discuss his views on the questionnaire. He asked that a few small changes be made. These included:
1. The alteration of the word 'spouse' to 'partner' (Q.7)
2. The inclusion of 'status epilepticus' with the types of epilepsy (Q.32)
3. The inclusion of options (e.g. G.P./Doctor, Neurologist Paediatrician, Other) in the question regarding who carried out the first general assessment/examination (Q.23)
4. The inclusion of a question that asked parents if they were aware that special exam conditions are made available by the Department of Education for children with epilepsy (Q.90)
5. The inclusion of 'mainstream school with special facilities' as an option for the type of school that parents felt would best provide for their child's specific needs. He also asked that the option 'special school for children with mental handicap' be changed to 'special school for children with learning difficulties' and be placed as a last option in the question (Q.109)
6. The inclusion of 'go onto a training course' in the options that described parents' expectations for their child in the future (Q.110)

The Chief Executive thought that the questionnaire was very worthwhile, but expressed reservations about its length. He asked if he could include a letter to the parents stressing the importance of the questionnaire and advising them that their area representative of Brainwave, the Irish Epilepsy Association would be available to assist them if they had difficulties with any part of it (Appendix 5). He requested that the above alterations be made before returning it to him. It was then to be given to a neurologist at the Children's Hospital, Temple Street and to a senior clinical neuropsychologist at Beaumont Hospital for their opinions. The alterations were made and the questionnaire was returned to Brainwave, the Irish Epilepsy Association on Thursday 18th March 1999. The researcher was contacted over a week later (Tuesday 30th March 1999) with the following further recommendations:

Comments from the Clinical Neuropsychologist at Beaumont Hospital:
1. The removal of the words 'adversely affected the child' from the question relating to medication or drugs that the mother might have taken during the pregnancy, as she felt it may be confusing for the respondent (Q.14)
2. The alteration of the option 'brain meninges' to 'brain meningitis' because she felt that parents might be more familiar with that term (Q.15)
3. Simplification of the question relating to the first clinical assessment, as parents may be unclear about general medical assessment versus clinical assessment (Q.23/24)
4. The removal of one of the questions about how their child's condition was first explained, as she thought there was an overlap (Q.27/28)
5. The inclusion of the option to tick any of the emotions felt when they first heard the diagnosis (Q.30)
6. The replacement of the word 'self-esteem' with 'confidence' (Q.107)
7. The inclusion of a positive option regarding how the teacher relates to their child (Q.87)
8. The inclusion of a positive option regarding how their child feels about having epilepsy (Q.92)

9. The alteration of 'partial or focal epilepsy' to 'temporal lobe or focal epilepsy', because she felt that parents might not be familiar with the former term (Q.32)
10. The inclusion of hyperactivity as a behaviour-related reaction to medication (Q.55)
11. The correction of a typographical error in Q.31

She also commented that it would be a very valuable piece of work.

Comments from the Consultant Paediatric Neurologist at the Children's Hospital, Temple Street.
He commented on the length of the questionnaire, but felt that it was clearly comprehensive and well thought-out. He made the following recommendations:
1. He asked that a question regarding frequency of seizures be included.
2. He advised that a question asking whether the child is presently experiencing any of the listed side effects be added.
3. He warned about being cautious in presenting information in relation to parents' recollections regarding birth complications because parental information about birth complications is often faulty and may be exaggerated by retrospection, in light of subsequent problems.
4. He also advised on the presentation of data regarding parents' recollections about how much they were told, or how much was explained by physicians, as it is well known that parents often remember incorrectly or take a more pessimistic view than that presented.

Parents'Opinions/Responses
The questionnaire was also sent to parents of five children with epilepsy:
• a girl of 18 who developed epilepsy at 11 years of age
• a girl of 11 who developed epilepsy at eight
• a girl who had epilepsy from birth and was placed in a special school at 7, despite having no other condition
• a boy of nine who was diagnosed in July 1997
• a boy of 16 who has had epilepsy since he was two years of age

Their responses showed that a number of the questions needed some small alterations. These included:
1. Underlining of the word 'pregnancy' in question 12, because one of the parents wrote about difficulties during birth. (Q.12)
2. The inclusion of the option 'none' in the question relating to the areas in which advice was given to the parents on how to manage their child. (Q.57)
3. The inclusion of the option 'none of these' in the question regarding activities which their child's epilepsy makes them reluctant to do. (Q. 103)

The above changes were made by Wednesday 31st March 1999 and a meeting with the Chief Executive of Brainwave, the Irish Epilepsy Association, was held on Thursday 1st April 1999 for a final review of the questionnaire and introductory letters.

7.7   DATA COLLECTION
A total of 139 questionnaires, accompanied by a letter from the researcher (Appendix 6) and the Chief Executive of Brainwave, describing the nature and purpose of the enquiry, were distributed in April 1999. A follow up letter, telephone calls and two notices in Epilepsy News, Brainwave's Newsletter (Appendix 7), secured the return of 65 (47%) completed questionnaires.

In view of the length of the questionnaire and the level of medical awareness required to complete it, a response rate of 47% was deemed extremely good. Given the emotional climate which many of the questions may have induced in respondents, and the fact that the sheer day-to-day management of their child's condition proves very difficult, the response rate was very high. The psychological affect that the questionnaire may have had on some parents must also be appreciated, as it highlighted the full implications of the condition. This was clearly illustrated by a parent, who commented that "Explaining our feelings etc. was particularly painful but this survey can only help our little girl." Due to the lack of precise information concerning the basis upon which the sample was nominated, it was not possible to draw any defensible conclusions about the characteristics of non-respondents.

7.8   DATA ANALYSIS

Data obtained from the questionnaires was coded manually in order to facilitate entry and analysis using SPSS programme, version 8.0 (Microsoft Works, 1997).   Qualitative information gleaned from open-ended questions, which reflected significant areas of concern for parents of children with epilepsy, was subjected to a content analysis.   A number of these individual parental comments relating to specific items are reported in the results.

7.9   FUNDING

A bursary of five hundred pounds for educational research was received from the Irish National Teacher's Organisation, under their Grant for Educational Research Scheme in January 1999. Brainwave, the Irish Epilepsy Association also provided financial assistance by mailing the questionnaires.   A Millennium Scholarship of two thousand pounds, in support of the research, was awarded by the Church of Ireland College of Education, in November 2000.

7.10 LIMITATIONS OF THE STUDY

It proved very difficult for professionals involved in State Departments of Health and Education and Science to furnish the researcher with data regarding the number of school-going children with epilepsy in the Republic of Ireland.   Following numerous telephone calls to various departments in the Department of Education and Science, the Department of Health and Children and each Health Board, it became apparent that no reliable statistics concerning the incidence of epilepsy within the school-going population were available.

According to Mr. Brian Cowen T.D., Minister for Health and Children, the establishment and maintenance of records arising from the screening programmes run by the Health Boards in schools, is a matter solely for each Health Board (Appendix 8).   However, from the replies received from each Health Board (Appendix 9), it appeared that no statistics on epilepsy have ever been compiled from the Schools' Health Screening Service.   The researcher was told that, in order to ascertain the number of children with epilepsy in each district, the records would have to be counted manually.   According to the Programme Manager of the North Western Health Board, the Screening Service in his area tends to focus on the "detection of new, previously undetected problems….Information (on childhood epilepsy) would be collected as part of the child's medical history, but this would be incomplete."   Similarly, the Medical Officer in the North Eastern Health Board replied that "the schools' screening programme in Co. Meath has concentrated on the detection of clinically significant conditions which the parents may be unaware of."   The Director of Public Health for the Southern Health Board responded that "information systems are not sufficiently developed within Health Boards to provide information that is reliable, valid and accurate without considerable resource investment which is not available."   The responses from the Health Boards clearly show that the establishment of such a database is crucial, if only because the lack of regular, carefully co-ordinated studies of the aetiology and prevalence rate of epilepsy among the Irish adult and child population makes it virtually impossible to establish their medical and educational needs.

Therefore, the researcher was entirely dependent on Brainwave, the Irish Epilepsy Association, a voluntary organisation, and its members for assistance in conducting substantive research in this area.   Consequently, it cannot be claimed that the views reported in this survey are representative of all parents of children with epilepsy in Ireland since the response sample consisted only of parents who joined Brainwave as a means of learning more about their child's condition.   While valuable information was gleaned using a questionnaire as a method of data collection, the researcher would have liked to interview some of the parents who gave detailed commentaries on their experiences with both medical and educational professionals.   Due to time constraints this was not possible.

As a supplementary aspect of the study, the researcher intended to conduct interviews with principals of both a mainstream and special school in order to establish how epilepsy is catered for by the Department of Education, Northern Ireland. Interviews were deemed unnecessary as telephone conversations with two principals and the special education officers in the five Education and Library Boards provided the researcher with adequate information.

7.11 CONCLUSION

In order to gain a perspective on the general applicability and relevance of the findings, the study concluded with a structured interview with the Chief Executive of Brainwave, the Irish Epilepsy Association in May 2000. In particular, the interview sought to establish the feasibility of the recommendations, the extent to which they applied to Brainwave as an organisation, and their specific relevance to the general improvement of the medical and educational provision for children with epilepsy the Republic of Ireland. Following the interview, a copy of the transcribed dialogue was submitted to the Chief Executive of Brainwave, the Irish Epilepsy Association, for his perusal in order that any necessary clarifications or extensions could be made.

Despite the constraints under which this research was conducted, the empirical study proved to be successful in achieving its aims. Parents who participated in the study were committed and helpful, and, most significantly, the resulting information provided the first database on children with epilepsy in the Republic of Ireland and on their parents' experiences of the medical and educational support services in the State.

CHAPTER EIGHT

PARENTS' OPINIONS ON AND EXPERIENCES OF PROVISION FOR CHILDREN WITH EPILEPSY

FIGURE 1: Children's Age Groups by Gender

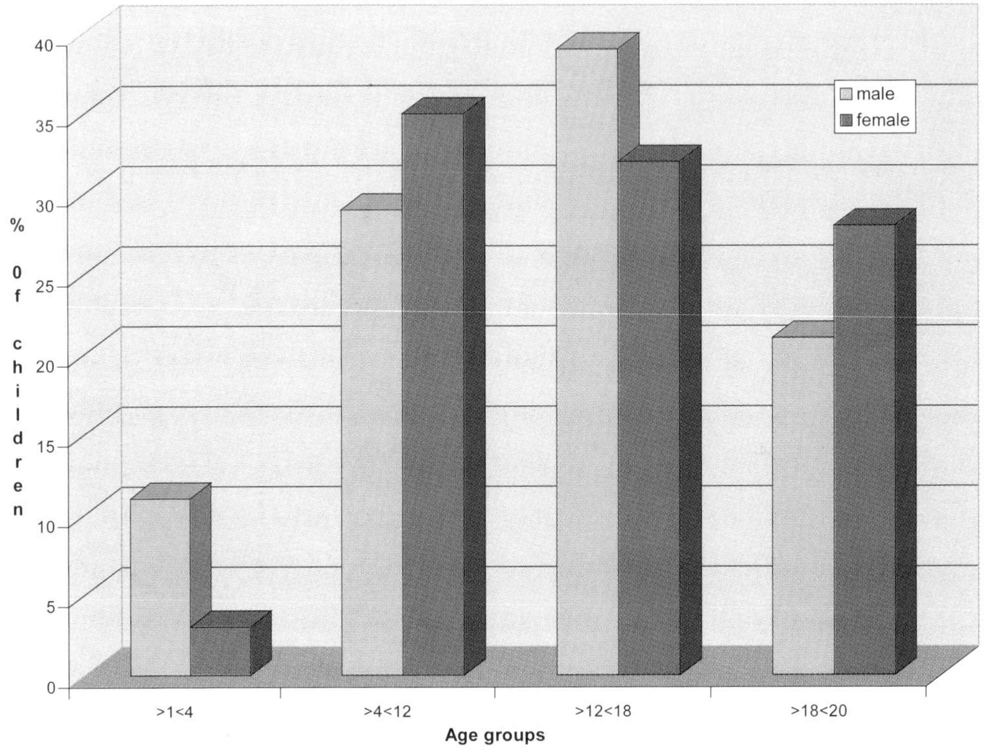

8.1   INTRODUCTION

In order to ascertain the views of parents on provision for children with epilepsy in the Republic of Ireland, a sample of parents drawn by the Irish Epilepsy Association was surveyed through a detailed postal questionnaire devised by the researcher (Appendix 4).   The questionnaire contained eight sections, each section addressing specific areas.

The responses of parents are presented in this chapter under headings similar to those used in the questionnaire. Some of the parental comments are also included where it is considered that these added important contextual information to the results.

8.2   BACKGROUND DETAILS
8.2.1 Age and Gender
Figure 1 shows that. of the children represented in the survey, 6% (n=4) were in the >1<4 age group; 32% (n=21) were in the >4<12 age group; 35% (n=23) were in the >12<18 age group and 26% (n=17) were in the >18<20 age group. Forty three per cent (n=28) of the children were male, while 57% (n=37) were female.

8.2.2 Respondent's Relationship to Child
Figure 2 shows that of those who completed the questionnaire, 89% (n=58) of the respondents were the mothers and 11% (n=7) the fathers of the children represented in the study.

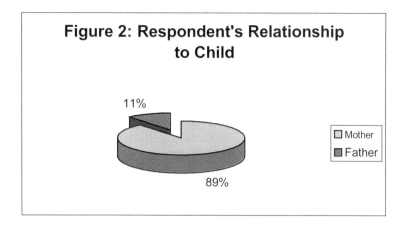

Figure 2: Respondent's Relationship to Child

11%

89%

☐ Mother
☑ Father

8.2.3 Marital Situation

Figure 3 illustrates that 91% (n=59) of the children surveyed were living with both their natural parents; 1% (n=1) had one parent deceased and 8% (n=5) had parents who were separated. The National Child Development Study (NCDS) in Britain found that, as a group, one-parent families of children with epilepsy were over-represented and that divorce and death were more common than expected (Ross et al., 1980). Betts et al. (1993) also contend that epilepsy can be a focus for conflict, resulting in higher rates of separation and divorce. The level of separation in this study was very low. This may possibly be due to the fact that divorce is a relatively recent phenomenon in Ireland

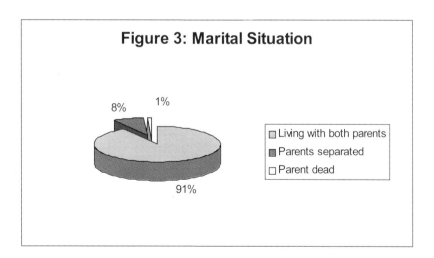

Figure 3: Marital Situation

8%   1%

91%

☐ Living with both parents
☑ Parents separated
☐ Parent dead

8.2.4 Number of Children in Family

Figure 4 illustrates the number of children in the family. Of the families surveyed, 11% (n=7) had one child; 26% (n=17) had two children; 31% (n=20) had three children. Twenty five per cent (n=16) of families had four children; 1% (n=1) had five children; 3% (n=2) had six children and 3% (n=2) had seven children.

FIGURE 4: Number of Children in Family

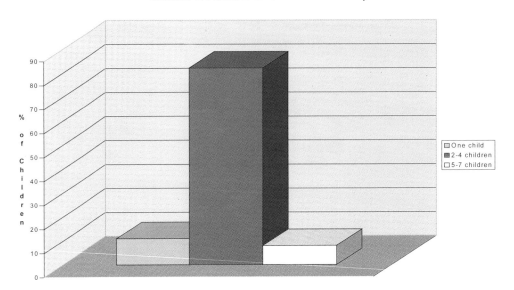

FIGURE 6: Respondents' and Partners' Levels of Education

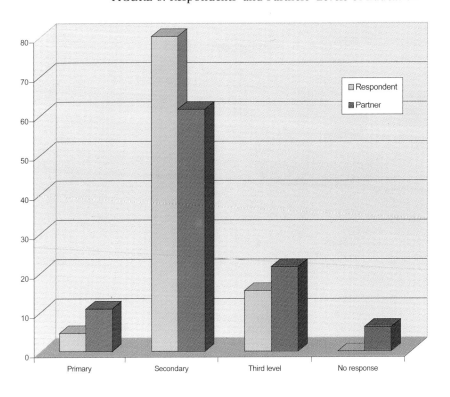

8.2.5 Position in Family

Figure 5 illustrates the children's position in the family. In 34% (n=22) of cases, the children sampled were the eldest in their family; 26% (n=17) were in the middle; 29% (n=19) were the youngest, while 11% (n=7) were "only children".

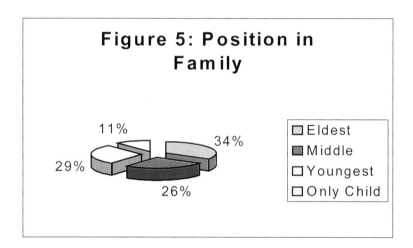

8.2.6 Parents' Levels of Education

Figure 6 illustrates the parents' levels of education. Five per cent (n=3) of the respondents completed primary school only, 80% (n=52) completed primary and secondary schooling while 15% (n=10) completed primary, secondary and third level education.

Of the respondents' partners, 11% (n=7) attended primary only, 62% (n=40) completed primary and secondary, 22% (n=14) completed primary, secondary and third level education. Six per cent (n=4) gave no response but the researcher believes that this may due to the fact that they did not complete primary level education, as the question asked the respondent to tick the levels of education completed. Analysis of their occupations showed that they were unemployed.

8.3   INCIDENCE OF EPILEPSY AMONG FAMILY MEMBERS

Table 1 illustrates the incidence of epilepsy among family members. Of the families surveyed, 8% (n=5) of the mothers and 5% (n=3) of the fathers also had epilepsy. Five per cent (n=3) of the maternal grandmothers and 3% (n=2) of the paternal grandmothers had epilepsy. None of the maternal grandfathers were reported to have epilepsy but 2% (n=1) of the paternal grandfathers did. Two per cent (n=1) of maternal aunts and 3% (n=2) of paternal aunts were reported to have epilepsy. Three per cent (n=2) of maternal uncles and 5% (n=3) of paternal uncles had epilepsy. Fourteen per cent (n=9) of maternal cousins and 12% (n=8) of paternal cousins were also reported to have epilepsy.

Table 1: Incidence of Epilepsy Among Family Members

Relationship to Child	N	%
Maternal cousins	9	13.8
Paternal cousins	8	12.3
Mother	5	7.7
Siblings	4	6.2
Father	3	4.6
Maternal Grandmother	3	4.6
Paternal Uncles	3	4.6
Paternal Grandmother	2	3.1
Paternal Aunts	2	3.1
Maternal Uncles	2	3.1
Paternal Grandfather	1	1.5
Maternal Aunts	1	1.5
Maternal Grandfather	0	0
Total	**43**	**66.1**

The prediction of risks for the offspring of individuals who have epilepsy depends on the nature of the parental epilepsy. According to McMenamin and O'Connor Bird (1997), some forms of epilepsy such as absence seizures, generalised tonic-clonic seizures of the idiopathic variety and photosensitive epilepsy have a strong hereditary basis. However, it is not known what type of epilepsy the parents in this sample had. Hauser and Anderson (1986) state that the overall incidence of seizures in the offspring when one parent is affected is about four per cent, but when both parents are affected it rises to ten per cent or more. However, O'Donohue (1985) reports that where both parents have epilepsy, it is approximately 25%.

Six per cent (n=4) of the children in the sample had a sibling with epilepsy.

Parental Description of Siblings' Epilepsy
The parents gave the following descriptions regarding three of the four children:
- The youngest child is female and has epilepsy since day two of life. Now at sixteen months old she is still having seizures, even though on medication she has developed very slowly.
- The other child has suffered absent spells of one or two seconds duration, plus has had seizures with high temperatures.
- Had yearly seizure.

As the type of epilepsy the siblings had was not specified, it is not possible to comment on its incidence among them. According to O'Donohue (1994), the incidence of epilepsy among siblings depends on the type of epilepsy within their family.

8.4 PREGNANCY AND BIRTH CIRCUMSTANCES
8.4.1 Circumstances During Pregnancy
Complications cited are summarised in Table 2. Complications during pregnancy were reported by 20% (n=13) of the sample. They included: preclampsia, toxaemia, gestational diabetes, premature birth, near death of mother/baby, detachment of placenta at seven months, removal of the gall bladder and one case of multiple complications including high blood pressure, toxaemia and premature birth.

Table 2: Complications During Pregnancy

Reported Complications	N	%
Premature Birth	3	4.6
Preclampsia	2	3.1
Placenta Detached	2	3.1
Toxaemia	1	1.5
Gestational Diabetes	1	1.5
Mother/Baby nearly died	1	1.5
Multiple Complications*	1	1.5
Threatened spontaneous abortion	1	1.5
Gall Bladder Removed	1	1.5
Total	13	19.8

*High blood pressure/toxaemia, premature baby

When comparing risk factors in healthy children and children with epilepsy, Rantakallio and von Wendt (1986) found that prenatal factors formed the highest risks. In children with epilepsy, prenatal causes of epilepsy could be found in 9% of children, perinatal causes in 18% and postnatal causes in 16%. However, prematurity and low birth weight did not seem to be important risk factors.

Figure 7 shows the number of mothers who smoked or drank during pregnancy. Fifty eight per cent (n=38) of the mothers neither drank or smoked during their pregnancy. Of the 42% (n=27) who did, 20% (n=13) smoked, 17% (n–11) drank and 5% (n=3) both smoked and drank.

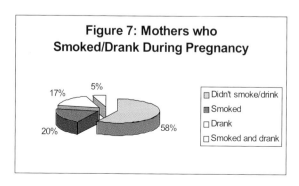

Figure 7: Mothers who Smoked/Drank During Pregnancy

17% 5%
20% 58%

- □ Didn't smoke/drink
- ■ Smoked
- □ Drank
- □ Smoked and drank

Eighty six per cent (n=56) of the mothers took no medication during pregnancy (see Figure 8). Of the 14% (n=9) who did, 5% (n=3) took anti-epileptic medication, 3% (n=2) took asthma medication, 1.5% (n=1) took painkillers, 1.5% (n=1) took Detendox tablets prescribed by a doctor for vomiting and 1.5% (n=1) took Clonamox, an antibiotic.

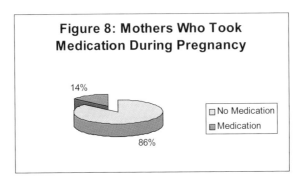

8.4.2 Circumstances at Birth

Table 3 shows the reported complications during birth. Birth complications were reported by 40% (n=26) of the sample. Twenty five per cent (n=16) of the mothers had prolonged labour; 1.5% (n=1) of the children received injury to the head; 9% (n=6) of the mothers reported prolonged delivery; 19% (n=12) had a forceps delivery and 6% (n=4) of the children had lack of oxygen during the birth. Many of the mothers reported a combination of the above complications.

Twenty per cent (n=13) also reported other birth complications. These included: the cord being wrapped around the baby's neck when born 1.5% (n=1); the waters being inhaled by the baby 1.5% (n=1); baby not breathing when born/vacuum delivery 3%(n=2); cord wrapped around neck and the waters inhaled 1.5% (n=1); baby and mother in distress during birth 5% (n=3); caesarian section 6% (n=4); baby infected by dirty tube in incubator 1.5% (n=1).

Table 3: Birth Complications

Birth Complications	N	%
Prolonged Labour	16	24.6
Forceps Delivery	12	18.5
Prolonged Delivery	6	9.2
Lack of Oxygen During Birth	4	6.2
Caesarian Section	4	6.2
Baby/Mother in Distress During Birth	3	4.6
Baby Not Breathing/Vacuum Delivery	2	3.1
Head Injury	1	1.5
Cord Wrapped Around Neck	1	1.5
Waters Inhaled By Baby	1	1.5
Cord Wrapped Around Neck/Waters Inhaled	1	1.5
Baby Infected By Dirty Incubator Tube	1	1.5
Total	52	79.9

In studies from Iceland (Gudmundsson, 1986) and Norway (Krohn, 1961), difficulties in delivery were regarded as constituting the most important aetiological factor. O'Connor *et al.* (1992) and McMenamin and O'Connor Bird (1997) also state that post-traumatic epilepsy can occur as a result of a severe head trauma which causes direct injury to the brain.

8.4.3 Medical Conditions at Birth

Table 4 summarises the medical conditions at birth. Nine per cent (n=6) of the total sample had epilepsy from birth. Fourteen per cent (n=9) also reported other medical conditions which included: cerebral palsy, Down's Syndrome, hydrocephalus, asthma, congenital adrenal hyperplasia, respiratory distress syndrome, dislocated shoulder bone and "floppiness at birth".

Table 4: Medical Conditions at Birth

Medical Condition	N	%
Hydrocephalus	2	3.1
Cerebral Palsy	1	1.5
Down's Syndrome	1	1.5
Asthma	1	1.5
Floppiness at Birth	1	1.5
Congenital Adrenal Hyperplasia	1	1.5
Respiratory Distress Syndrome	1	1.5
Dislocated Shoulder Bone	1	1.5
Total	9	13.6

McKusick (1983) comments that there are over 100 single gene disorders which may have epilepsy as a symptom. O'Donohue (1994) also states that seizures may occur in clinical syndromes caused by chromosomal anomalies such as Down's Syndrome. According to Rocca *et al.* (1987a), epilepsy is significantly more common among persons with cerebral palsy, head trauma and viral encephalitis.

8.5   DEVELOPMENTAL HISTORY

Table 5 summarises parents' satisfaction with their child's general development. The most significant developmental problem was in the area of concentration, which 21% (n=14) of parents reported as being non-satisfactory. General alertness (11%; n=7) and behaviour (12%; n=8) were also reported to be areas of developmental concern. Although language understanding (6%; n=4) was not regarded as a significant problem, speech, both articulation (15%; n=10) and expression (14%; n=9), were noted as not being satisfactory. Hearing and vision were reported as being non-satisfactory in 12% (n=8) and 15% (n=10) of cases respectively. Physical co-ordination was reported as being non-satisfactory by 11% (n=7) of parents. Sociability and ability to relate to others were regarded as developmental problems in only 9% (n=6) of cases.

Table 5: Parents' Satisfaction with Child's General Development

Aspect of Development	Unsatisfactory
Concentration	21.5 (n=14)
Vision	15.4 (n=10)
Speech (articulation)	15.4 (n=10)
Language-Expression	13.8 (n=9)
Behaviour	12.3 (n=8)
Hearing	12.3 (n=8)
General Alertness	10.8 (n=7)
Physical Co-ordination	10.8 (n=7)
Ability to Relate to Others	9.3 (n=6)
Language Understanding	6.2 (n=4)

Parents' Comments Regarding Child's Development
The following are the comments made by some of the parents regarding their child's development:
- Development was normal until the seizures began
- I feel that they, as in doctors and specialists, were poor in relating to his speech and language problems. Even now he suffers from hearing and understanding difficulties.
- He developed deafness in one ear (right) at age four due to mumps.
- No eyesight in one eye, 25% in other
- Suffered with hearing from a young age
- Developed Ocular Myasthenia Gravis at two years
- X is a hyperactive child- he can be really very difficult
- X had very bad ear infections and had grommets inserted twice
- Squint in left eye-had to wear glasses at 18 months
- Child is first grandchild-so was a loner-spent a lot of time day dreaming or so we thought, now it turns out she was having minor fits
- She has had a lot of behavioural problems since early childhood and has found it very difficult to relate to her peers.
- Showing signs of strange behaviour problems-obsessive, and emotional problems
- Was a very quiet child–is now easily annoyed and agitated
- The child seemed to have difficulty in expressing herself verbally. She seemed to be thinking ahead of herself.
- All of the above were very satisfactory until her first epileptic seizure
- Problems only arose after diagnosis at approximately age five

Table 6: Particular Behaviours That Caused Initial Parental Concern

Particular Behaviours	N	%
Had a seizure	25	38.5
Twitches	9	13.8
Shaking/Jerking	5	7.7
Trances	4	6.2
Febrile convulsions	3	4.6
Unusual Behaviour	3	4.6
Dizzy spell	2	3.1
Trances /Unusual head and body movements	2	3.1
Aggressive behaviour and disturbed sleep patterns	2	3.1
Behavioural changes/dropping items	2	3.1
Dropping to ground continuously	1	1.5
Leg cramps and crying at night	1	1.5
Crying continuously	1	1.5
Swelling of fontanelle	1	1.5
Choking sensations	1	1.5
Burning sensation in leg	1	1.5
Migraine headaches	1	1.5
Total	**64**	**98.3**

Missing Cases: 1

The data indicates that some of the children experienced difficulties in the area of concentration and speech. However, many of the parents commented that the child's early development was satisfactory until the first seizure occurred.

8.6   INITIAL REFERRAL AND DIAGNOSIS
8.6.1 Early Symptomatology of Epilepsy

Table 6 summarises the various behaviours that caused initial parental concern. In 5% (n=3) of cases, parents suspected that something was wrong with their child at birth. In 38% (n=25) of cases, there were no particular behaviours or warning signs prior to the first seizure. In 14% (n=9) of cases, the characteristic which caused initial parental concern was the presence of twitches. Other particular behaviours which made the parents suspect something was wrong included: febrile convulsions (5%; n=3); shaking and jerking (8%; n=5); dizzy spell (3%; n=2); trances (6%; n=4); dropping to the ground continuously (1.5%; n=1); trances and unusual head and body movements (3%; n=2); leg cramps and crying at night (1.5%; n=1); aggressive behaviour and disturbed sleep patterns (3%; n=2); crying continuously (1.5%; n=1); swelling of fontanelle (1.5%; n=1); behavioural changes and dropping items (3%; n=2); choking sensations (1.5%; n=1); unusual behaviour (5%; n=3); burning sensation in leg (1.5%; n=1) and migraine headaches (1.5%; n=1).

In 3% (n=2) of cases, the parents did not suspect that their child had epilepsy. For the other parents, the age-range at which epilepsy was suspected varied from one day old to nearly 18 years old.

Table 7 shows that in 20% (n=13) of cases, it was the parents themselves that suggested their child might have epilepsy. However, for most of the parents it was a professional, such as their doctor (41.5%; n=27), paediatrician (23.1%; n=15), neurologist (3.1%; n=2), paediatrician and neurologist (1.5%; n=1) or nurse (3.1%; n=2), who suggested that their child had epilepsy. For 4.6% (n=3) it was a combination of the parent, family friend and doctor that made the suggestion. In two cases, it was either a relative (1.5%; n=1) or a friend (1.5%; n=1).

Table 7: Person Who Suggested Child Had Epilepsy

Person	N	%
Doctor	27	41.5
Paediatrician	15	23.1
Parent	13	20.0
Parent/friend/doctor	3	4.6
Nurse	2	3.1
Neurologist	2	3.1
Paediatrician/Neurologist	1	1.5
Relative	1	1.5
Friend	1	1.5
Total	65	100

Figure 9 illustrates the type of medical professional who carried out the first general examination.

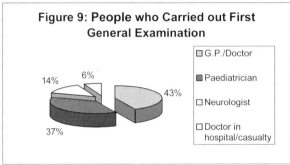

In 43% (n=28) of cases, it was the family doctor who carried out the first general medical examination. Other professionals reported to have examined the child included: paediatricians (37%; n=24); neurologists (14%; n=9) and doctors in the casualty department of their local hospital (6%; n=4).

Table 8: Hospitals Where Neurologist Was Attended

Hospital	N	%
Did not attend one	11	16.8
Crumlin Hospital	26	40.0
Temple Street Hospital	10	15.4
Beaumont Hospital	3	4.6
St. Vincent's Hospital	3	4.6
St. James' Hospital	2	3.1
Rotunda Hospital	1	1.5
Adelaide Hospital	1	1.5
Cork Hospital	6	9.2
Total	63	96.8

Missing Cases: 2

Analysis of the early diagnosis of the child's epilepsy suggests that in 57% (n=37) of cases, the parents suspected that something was wrong with their child because of particular behaviours such as shaking and jerking or trances. However, in 38% (n=25) of cases there were no particular warning signs prior to the first seizure. For most of the parents (77%; n=50), it was a medical professional, such as a doctor or a paediatrician, who suggested that their child had epilepsy. In 43% (=28) of cases, it was the family doctor who carried out the first general medical examination.

8.6.2 Initial Referral

Eighty per cent (n=52) of parents reported that their child attended a neurologist, while in 17% (n=11) of cases the child did not attend a neurologist.

Table 8 lists the hospitals where neurologists were attended. Forty per cent (n=26) reported that they attended a neurologist in Crumlin Children's Hospital; 15.4% (n=10) attended Temple Street Children's Hospital; 4.6% (n=3) attended St. Vincent's Hospital; 4.6% (n=3) attended Beaumont Hospital; 3.1% (n=2) attended St. James' Hospital; 1.5% (n=1) attended the Rotunda Hospital; 1.5% (n=1) attended the Adelaide Hospital and 9.2% (n=6) attended a hospital in Cork.

Table 9 shows the specific waiting periods for referral to a specialist. In 6% (n=4) of cases, there was no referral waiting period because the child was examined following birth. Fifteen per cent (n=10) of the children were seen straight away when hospitalised following a seizure. In 11% (n=7) of cases, the parents reported that they attended a specialist privately and therefore, had a relatively short waiting period. For the remaining parents who attended a specialist publicly, the waiting period varied from four days to 360 days. One parent reported that she had waited six years for a referral to a specialist. This was because her doctor did not believe that there was anything wrong with her child and would not refer her. In 10.8% (n=7) of cases, no waiting period was reported, either because the parents could not remember it or because their child was referred immediately.

Table 9: Length Waiting for a Referral to a Specialist

Number of Days	Frequency	%
4	1	1.5
7	2	3.1
11	1	1.5
14	7	10.8
21	3	4.6
28	3	4.6
30	3	4.6
35	1	1.5
42	3	4.6
60	3	4.6
90	4	6.2
120	1	1.5
180	1	1.5
270	1	1.5
360	1	1.5
2190	1	1.5
Total	**36**	**55.1**

Analysis of the initial referral procedures shows that a large percentage (83%; n=54) of the children attended a neurologist. Although the sample was geographically dispersed across the country, 71% (n=46) of the children attended a neurologist in Dublin. In 6% (n=4) of cases, there was no waiting period because the children were examined following birth. However, of the 54% (n=35) of parents who attended a specialist publicly, their waiting period ranged from four days to 360 days.

8.6.3 Diagnosis Of Other Medical Conditions

Table 10 summarises other medical conditions which were diagnosed. Ninety three per cent (n=60) of the children had no other medical condition. Other conditions which were diagnosed included: cerebral palsy (1.5%; n=1); cerebral palsy and speech impairment (1.5%; n=1); Down's Syndrome (1.5%; n=1); speech impairment (1.5%; n=1) and brain not fully developed (1.5%; n=1).

Table 10: Other Medical Conditions

Condition	N	%
Cerebral Palsy	1	1.5
C.Palsy/Speech Impairm.	1	1.5
Down's Syndrome	1	1.5
Speech Impairment	1	1.5
Brain not fully developed	1	1.5
Total	**5**	**7.5**

8.6.4 Diagnosis of Epilepsy

As shown in Table 11, the description of the child's condition was conveyed to parents in various ways. In 74% (n=48) of cases, the word epilepsy was used when the doctor or specialist was telling the parents of their child's condition. However, in 25% (n=16) of cases the child's condition was conveyed in such a way that the parents were unclear about the diagnosis, as the word epilepsy was not used. The other terms used included: drop attacks/seizures/fits/turns (6.2%; n=4); episodes (6.2%; n=4); petit mal (4.6%; n=3); jitters (1.5%; n=1); benign focal seizures (1.5%; n=1); epileptiform seizure (1.5%; n=1) and fever convulsions (1.5%; n=1). In one case (1.5%; n=1), the condition was described as hormonal and the parents were told it was probably age-related, as the boy was 13 years and 9 months. The parents did not realise that their child had epilepsy until a later consultation. One child's parents were told that they were first time parents and the child only had the jitters.

Table 11: Specialists' Descriptions of Child's Condition

Description	N	%
Epilepsy	48	74.0
Drop attacks/seizures/fits	4	6.2
Episodes	4	6.2
Petit mal	3	4.6
Jitters	1	1.5
Hormonal	1	1.5
Benign focal seizures	1	1.5
Epileptiform seizure	1	1.5
Fever convulsions	1	1.5
Total	64	98.5

Missing case:1

The suggested causes of epilepsy are listed in Table 12. In 85% (n=55) of cases, there was no cause suggested for the child's epilepsy. Difficult birth circumstances was suggested for 3% (n=2) of cases. Other suggested causes included: scar on mesial lobe (1.5%; n=1); related to cerebral palsy (1.5%; n=1); insufficient sleep (1.5%; n=1); calcification of skull (1.5%; n=1); flashing computer screen (3%; n=2); 3 in 1 injection (1.5%; n=1) and migraine headaches (1.5%; n=1).

Table 12: Suggested Causes of Epilepsy

Suggested Cause	N	%
None Given	55	84.6
Difficult Birth	2	3.1
Scar on Mesial Lobe	1	1.5
Computer Screen	2	3.1
Insufficient Sleep	1	1.5
Related to Cerebral Palsy	1	1.5
Calcification of skull	1	1.5
3 in 1 injection	1	1.5
Migraine	1	1.5
Total	65	100

In receiving the diagnosis of epilepsy, the reactions of the parents were mixed. These reactions are shown in Table 13. The majority of parents expressed reactions of anxiety (61.5%; n=40), shock (57%; n=37) and fear (51%, n=33). Other parents reported feeling sad (45%; n=29), confused (31%; n=20), and angry (23%; n=15). Some parents expressed feelings of disappointment (21.5%; n=14) and even guilt (18.5%; n=12). For 18.5% (n=12) of the parents, the diagnosis confirmed their suspicions that something was wrong and in doing so brought a sense of relief. One parent commented that she was relieved that the epilepsy hadn't been diagnosed as a brain tumor. Another parent was also relieved when the word epilepsy was finally used, since it was a label with which she could identify. Other reported emotions included: depression (11%; n=7); acceptance (15%; n=10); denial (5%; n=3); rejection (5%; n=3).

Table 13: Parents' Reactions to Diagnosis

Reaction	N	%
Anxiety	40	61.5
Shock	37	56.9
Fear	33	50.8
Sadness	29	44.6
Confusion	20	30.8
Anger	15	23.1
Disappointment	14	21.5
Guilt	12	18.5
Relief	12	18.5
Acceptance	10	15.4
Depression	7	10.8
Denial	3	4.6
Rejection	3	4.6

The parents' reactions to the diagnosis of their child's condition varied from anxiety to rejection and are similar to those reported by McGovern (1982), Wallace (1994), Pond (1981), Ward and Bower (1978) and Hall et al. (1997).

Table 14 illustrates the people that parents told about their child's diagnosis. A surprising 12% (n=8) of parents did not tell their partner that their child had been diagnosed with epilepsy. Analysis of the people whom individual parents told of the diagnosis of epilepsy showed that more relations on the mother's side than on the father's side of the family were told. For example, 69% (n=45) of maternal grandmothers were told, while only 51% (n=33) of paternal grandmothers were told. Fifty four per cent (n=35) of maternal grandfathers and 40% (n=26) of paternal grandfathers were told. Similarly, 85% (n=55) of maternal aunts and 68% (n=44) of paternal aunts were told. Seventy two per cent (n=47) of maternal uncles and 64% (n=42) of paternal uncles were told of the diagnosis. In 78.5% (n=51) of cases, maternal friends were told, while 61.5% (n=40) of paternal friends were told.

According to McGovern (1982), many fathers look on epilepsy in their child as a slur on their virility, particularly if the child is a son. This may explain why more relations on the mother's side than on the father's side of the family were told.

Table 15 illustrates other people whom the parents told of their child's condition. When asked if any people other than the above were informed 75% (n=49) of parents replied that they had not told anyone else. The parents who informed others listed the following: teachers (14%; n=9); club leaders (1.5%; n=1); siblings (3%; n=2); boss (1.5%; n=1); another mother of a child who also had epilepsy (3%; n=2) and doctor (1.5%; n=1).

Table 14: People Parents Told About Diagnosis

Person	N	%
Partner	57	87.7
Maternal Grandmother	45	69.2
Paternal Grandmother	33	50.8
Maternal Grandfather	35	53.8
Paternal Grandfather	26	40.0
Maternal Aunts	55	84.6
Paternal Aunts	44	67.7
Maternal Uncles	47	72.3
Paternal Uncles	42	64.6
Maternal Friends	51	78.5
Paternal Friends	40	61.5

Table 15: People Parents Told About Diagnosis

Person	N	%
No others	49	75.4
Teachers/School	9	13.8
Club Leaders	1	1.5
Siblings	2	3.1
Boss	1	1.5
Parent of Child with Epilepsy	2	3.1
Doctor/G.P.	1	1.5
Total	65	100

Table 16: Family Members' Reactions

Reaction	N	%
Understanding	13	20.0
Anxiety/Worry	9	13.8
Shock	7	10.8
Didn't Understand Condition	6	9.2
Fear/Concern	6	9.2
Shock/Denial	5	7.7
Shock/Relief	3	4.6
Denial	3	4.6
Devastated/Supportive	6	3.1
Sadness	2	3.1
Sadness/Worry	2	3.1
Disappointment	2	3.1
Fear	1	1.5
Anger	1	1.5
Fear/Anger	1	1.5
Relief/Happiness	1	1.5
Rejection	1	1.5
Total	65	100

Table 16 shows how the reactions of family members (e.g. partner, siblings, grandparents, relations) to the diagnosis of epilepsy varied from understanding to rejection. In 20% (n=13) of cases, parents reported that other family members were understanding about their child's condition. Other reactions included: anxiety/worry (14%; n=9); shock (11%; n=7); fear and concern (9%; n=6); "didn't understand the condition" (9%; n=6); shock and denial (8%; n=5); denial (5%; n=3); shock and relief (5%; n=3); devastated but supportive (3%; n=2); sadness (3%; n=2); sadness and worry (3%; n=2); disappointment (3%; n=2); anger (1.5%; n=1); fear (1.5%; n=1); fear and anger (1.5%; n=1); relief and happiness (1.5%; n=1) and rejection (1.5%; n=1).

Parental Comments Regarding Family Members' Reactions
Some of the comments regarding the reactions of family members included:
- A younger sister was hysterical that she would have to go through this epilepsy.
- Fear from children, anger from partner.
- With shock and sympathy

- Shock, and relief-with all the unexplained behaviour, it was an answer.
- Fear, sympathetic. Willingness to help. Wanted more information.
- Concerned, shocked and anxious.
- Denial-until diagnosis was confirmed.
- Shock at first because no other family member had epilepsy.
- Daughter's father expected me to be overprotective which caused a row.
- They hoped he would grow out of it and that it wouldn't effect his job/career prospects.
- With shock and then relief it was nothing more serious.
- Both our mothers had recently died and I thanked God they were not around to see X suffer.
- Epilepsy did not seem to be the problem but the mismanagement of X's condition by the } medical professionals was a huge problem.
- Disappointed, but coped.
- Partner was shocked and couldn't accept it.
- I think her older brother felt guilty because he used to lose patience with his sister when doing mathematics.
- As long as the seizures don't happen in public with them they don't mind.
- Sadness from the younger members, rejection from the older.
- They thought she would grow out of it.
- Devastated but very supportive and eager to learn about the condition.
- Very upset, confused. X's grandad had a heart attack within a couple of days of the fit-both were in hospital together.

8.6.5 Satisfaction With Referral And Diagnosis
When asked if they were satisfied with the way in which the doctor or specialist told them about their child's condition, 32% (n=21) reported that they were not satisfied. However, even the parents who reported that they were satisfied included some negative experiences and comments.

Parents' Reasons for Dissatisfaction with Referral and Diagnosis Procedures
- They did not use the word epilepsy. We were told some babies are born like this and they will grow out of it.
- We were not satisfied because he (the specialist) never really said he had epilepsy at the time of the diagnosis, and when my son was discharged from hospital two weeks later I was still in the dark as to what I should do to protect him.
- They did not explain. I thought they were very cold.
- Seemed to make quite light of it. Did not explain possible effects or consequences.
- Didn't tell us what to expect – that epilepsy comes at different times (night-day etc.).
- I was satisfied but it took them 39 seizures in six years to diagnose epilepsy. I also felt they expected me to know all about it in one day.
- I was not given enough information.
- He was very vague, using a lot of medical language, not very straightforward.
- His abrupt manner
- They weren't definite about the diagnosis and we got no information about the condition and even less on the medication – its side-effects, how it worked, its duration and who to contact if we had any worries or queries.
- Neurosurgeon told my son he had epilepsy and that he would just have to live with it. Very short and brief after waiting six months for full diagnosis. After waiting three hours for appointment in clinic we had three minutes with the specialist.
- Because we did not know about all aspects of her epilepsy i.e. behaviour as being part of epilepsy.
- Totally dissatisfied with X's (daughter's) entire treatment in X Hospital.
- I was told directly, which in a way was probably correct, but what I found most difficult was being told about all the things my child could not do, as opposed to what she could do, despite her condition. I found it most disturbing that all this was being discussed while my child sat there listening, and nothing seemed to be done to spare her feelings. I agree that she would need to know anyway, but at a later date when I felt the child could cope. The idea of a seven year old sitting there, listening to all sorts of medical jargon relating to herself and not understanding what it is all about, is worrying to me. I think there is a certain lack of sensitivity in the medical profession in this area. The paediatrician behaved in the same way. While I am all for explaining to a child what their illness entails, I feel there is a limit to the amount of

knowledge a seven year old needs.
- Nothing was discussed with us properly.
- Initially it was not fully explained to us.
- Was not explained in depth and we were not told where to get any information about it.
- I was not given enough information.
- Dissatisfied because the doctor never actually said the word "epilepsy".
- Dissatisfied with his abrupt manner.
- Seemed to make quite light of it. Did not explain possible effects or consequences.
- Was told he could be a "vegetable" and mildly autistic.

Many parents were unhappy with the way in which they told of their child's condition, simply because the specialist avoided the use of the word epilepsy, or they did not feel the condition was discussed in enough detail. When asked if they were confused by the terms used by the doctor or specialist, 40% (n=26) reported that they were.

Parents' Reasons for Confusion
- Yes, we were confused because, at the time we didn't know anything about the seizures until I got in contact with Brainwave.
- The explanations were too technical.
- The condition was not fully explained.
- Did not fully understand.
- Because we had never come into close contact with anyone with epilepsy we did not know anything about the condition.
- Confused by the types of seizures and whether temporal lobe was a seizure or just behaviour from temporal lobe.
- Did not know outcome of diagnosis.
- Confused because I had no prior knowledge of the condition.
- In the beginning I was told she had petit mal, which I was told was a very mild form of epilepsy but no, I didn't really understand what it meant.
- Unfamiliar with the condition.
- He was not very clear as to whether it was epilepsy and if so what type.
- I did not understand.
- The names for the different types of epilepsy are confusing.
- A little (confused) in that I still can't answer question 31 above. (The question relating to the type of epilepsy their child had)
- Yes, because they used every other word, but not epilepsy.

In 37% (n=24) of cases, the parents reported that they were not encouraged to ask questions about the diagnosis. When asked if they thought they were given enough clear explanations to help them understand and manage their child's condition at that point, 41% (n=27) of parents felt that they were not.

Parents' Reasons for Dissatisfaction with Lack of Information and Explanations
- We were sent home, told to give the child medication twice a day and come back for visits.
- No one told me anything e.g. What to do? Would they stop? Would he be able to grow normal?
- My son was given a pack of tablets and told to take them for the rest of his life.
- No directions. Learned to cope by own experience.
- Not told enough about epilepsy.
- They felt they were in charge and did not like me to ask too many questions and take up too much of their time.
- Doctors in clinic not helpful. Tests lost on two occasions.
- The professionals could not diagnose X's epilepsy for a long time. There was total mismanagement of X's medication and she almost died from an overdose of anti-convulsive drugs.
- Had to fight to get a doctor to see us.
- I was confused and needed a lot of questions to be answered.
- I was given very short answers to my questions and I felt that I needed more information.
- I had to go on the Internet to get all the information I needed. I wasn't given any addresses of organisations that could help.

Analysis of parents' satisfaction with referral and diagnosis procedures showed that many parents were unhappy about the manner in which they were treated, and the extent to which they were informed about their child's condition. Previous studies by Ward and Bower (1978), Hoare (1984), Andermann and Andermann (1992) de Boer (1995) and Tattenborn and Kramer (1992) have also reported parental dissatisfaction with both quantity and quality of information provided by medical professionals. According to Andermann and Andermann (1992), the better educated the person with epilepsy and their carers, the fewer the associated problems.

8.7   FOLLOW-UP SUPPORT AND COUNSELLING SERVICES
8.7.1 Counselling
For 78.5% (n=51) of the parents, no form of counselling or support facilities were recommended when their child was diagnosed with epilepsy.

Only 21.5% (n=14) of parents were recommended any support. Figure 10 illustrates the types of counselling and support services recommended. The recommendations given included contacting Brainwave (16.9%; n=11), contacting a neurology nurse (3%; n=2) and attending psychological counselling (1.5%; n=1). One parent commented that she was given the telephone number of the neurology nurse whom she could ring about any questions she might have.

The parents to whom Brainwave was recommended commented that they were either given leaflets about the organisation or given a contact number or name.

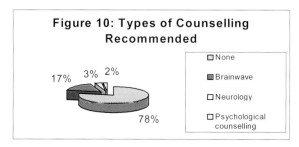

Figure 10: Types of Counselling Recommended

When asked if they had felt they needed counselling to help them deal with their child's epilepsy, 57% (n=37) reported that they did.

Parental Reasons for Needing Counselling
- It would have been nice to talk to some one when X was very ill.
- I did not understand why my son was having seizures and nobody was telling me any differently.
- At first I was devastated and felt alone. I spent eight months inside the house with my son afraid to take him outside.
- I needed counselling because I had never heard of this form of epilepsy (nocturnal) and don't know anybody whose child has it and I have not found anything written about it.
- I am very sad and depressed.
- Yes, for relief of worry.
- We got very frightened seeing X in a seizure.
- Did not know if I was coming or going with all the medication.
- Yes, because my doctor feels I have been traumatised by X's seizures.
- I needed counselling to enquire further about the condition.
- I had no experience of the condition and I felt very confused and scared and alone.
- To help cope with circumstances.
- I didn't know the first thing about the illness or its management, and as a family we were deeply concerned about our child's safety and future-what would it stop her doing?
- Sometimes the seizures were so severe that they frightened both my child and myself.
- I had no information and no idea of the reasons for this condition.
- Needed counselling for support and for information.
- We find life extremely difficult with regards management of the behavioural side.

- The whole experience of X's diagnosis was traumatic for all the family.
- When he was getting up to 30 seizures a day it was hard to come to terms with it.
- To help me accept epilepsy and deal with it, as it does not seem to be going away.
- We both needed counselling but it wasn't suggested to us.
- I had a fear of leaving her alone for even one minute, and started having panic attacks. I felt very isolated at times, as if no one understood.

Many of the parents wanted counselling as a means of obtaining more information, rather than helping them cope with the situation. Although 57% (n=37) of the parents had reported that they needed counselling, only 15% (n=10) had actually attended some form of counselling. Figure 11 illustrates the types of counselling attended. They included: Brainwave (8%; n=5); psychological counselling (6%; n=4) and a combination of Brainwave and psychological counselling (1.5%; n=1).

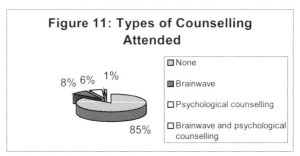

Figure 11: Types of Counselling Attended

Of the total sample of parents, 85% (n=56) did not attend counselling. Figure 12 illustrates the effectiveness of the counselling attended. Of those who did attend, 5% (n=3) found it very effective, 7% (n=4) found it effective and 3% (n=2) said it was not very effective.

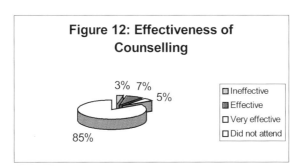

Figure 12: Effectiveness of Counselling

8.7.2 Other Information Which Would Have Helped
When asked if any other support or information would have helped with the particular difficulties which they were experiencing, 80% (n=52) replied that it would.

Suggested Parental Support and Information Which Would Have Helped

- Perhaps to talk to other families in the same situation.

- If there was someone, even a nurse or volunteer, to explain what was happening when your child is in hospital I think it would be helpful.

- Someone to talk to who was going through or had come out the other side of what I was going through.

- We knew nothing about epilepsy at the time and it seemed to us that neither did the doctor.

- Perhaps if a nurse had called to talk to us about epilepsy it would have helped us.

- Could have anticipated what might happen.

- More support and information regarding side-effects of anti-epileptic medication.
- Help to understand each kind of seizure.
- Support from other parents in the same situation i.e. Brainwave. More detailed information about the condition.
- Discussion with people in similar circumstances in my local area.
- To meet others who were going through same as me-especially where your child is concerned.
- Just simple basic information on the illness and its management.
- I feel the doctor should have given me leaflets with general information. I received these through my own efforts.
- Would have helped if someone had explained the medication side-effects and changes in lifestyle.
- More information on type of epilepsy and support from other parents with same difficulties. Family counselling.
- I strongly feel that professionals are not adequately trained in this area. They neither know or care less about patient and family care and support. I don't see a great deal has changed in 14 years.
- I feel that every doctor's surgery should display leaflets giving information on epilepsy, with contact numbers.
- It would have helped if they had mentioned Brainwave at an earlier stage.
- Help with dealing with seizures in public places.
- Meeting someone else's child that had exactly the same problems that we were experiencing with our child.
- More information about the medication was needed.
- Support groups
- We would like to have an epilepsy clinic locally that we could have gone to.
- Need to talk to others with the same condition.
- I think there should be immediate referral to a paediatric neurologist. General paediatricians do not have the same interest.
- Counselling –meeting others in the same circumstances.
- I would have liked to meet other parents at that time.
- We should have been informed about Brainwave through the hospital. It was just by chance that I read about Brainwave in our local newspaper.

The main support that many of the parents wanted was the opportunity to talk to other parents in the same situation.

The sources of information referred to by parents are listed in Table 17. In 88% (n=57) of cases, the parents looked for extra information about epilepsy. In 41.5% (n=27) of cases, parents contacted Brainwave for the extra information they required about their child's condition. Other sources of information included: Brainwave and medical books (18.5%; n=12); books (9%; n=6); Temple Street Hospital and their doctor (8%; n=5); Brainwave and hospital (6%; n=4); the Internet (1.5%; n=1). Three per cent (n=2) of parents did not get the information that they required about their child's condition. The neurological nursing staff in Temple Street Children's Hospital was also mentioned as sources by a number of parents. There was strong praise for Brainwave and their services, and the following comment illustrates the general gratitude felt by the parents who were aware of the organisation when their child was diagnosed: "They were at the other end of the phone at all times. They were great."

Table 17: Sources of Information

Source	N	%
Didn't Look for Information	8	12.3
Didn't Get Info. Sought	2	3.1
Brainwave	27	41.5
Brainwave/Books	12	18.5
Books	6	9.2
Temple Street Hosp./G.P.	5	7.7
Brainwave/Hospital	4	6.2
Internet	1	1.5
Total	65	100

Table 18: Types of Epilepsy

Type	N	%
Don't know	14	21.5
Tonic Clonic	17	26.2
Temporal Lobe/Focal E.	11	16.9
Tonic Clonic Absences/Drop and Jerk	6	9.2
Absences	5	7.7
Myoclonic or Jerk	4	6.2
Nocturnal	2	3.1
Akinetic or Drop Seizures	1	1.5
Frontal Lobe	1	1.5
Status Epilepticus/Tonic. Clonic/Absences/Temporal Lobe/Myoclonic	1	1.5
Partial	1	1.5
Tonic Clonic/Temporal Lobe/Focal	1	1.5
Tonic Clonic/Myoclonic	1	1.5
Total	65	100

Figure 13 illustrates how useful parents found the information they received. In 46% (n=30) of cases, parents rated it as very useful, 37% (n=24) as useful and 1.5% (n=1) as not very useful.

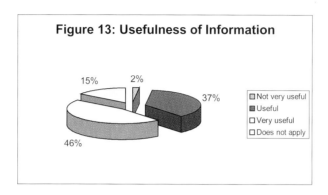

Figure 13: Usefulness of Information

- □ Not very useful
- ■ Useful
- □ Very useful
- □ Does not apply

8.8 MEDICAL ISSUES

8.8.1 Types of Epilepsy

The types of epilepsy reported by the parents in the sample are summarised in Table 18. Approximately 22% (n=14) of parents reported that they did not know what type of epilepsy their child had. Although a number of parents ticked a combination of the types given in the question, they also added in the comment, "I think!" The most frequently reported type of epilepsy was tonic clonic (26%; n=17) and temporal lobe or focal epilepsy (17%; n=11). Other types included: absences (8%; n=5); tonic clonic, absences and drop and jerk seizures (9%; n=6); myoclonic or jerk seizures (6%; n=4); nocturnal seizures (3%; n=2); status epilepticus, tonic clonic, absences, temporal lobe and myoclonic seizures (1.5%; n=1); partial seizures (1.5%; n=1); tonic clonic, temporal lobe, focal epilepsy (1.5%; n=1), tonic clonic and myoclonic (1.5%; n=1).

8.8.2 Frequency of Seizures

Table 19 shows the reported frequencies of seizures. In 11% (n=7) of cases, parents reported that their child had several seizures a day. Other reported frequencies included: one a day (1.5%; n=1); three to five a week (5%; n=3); one to two a week (5%; n=3); one to two a month (15%; n=10); less frequent than one a month (40%; n=26) and none now (23%; n=15). Those who reported that their child was not experiencing any seizures at present usually commented that it was because the medication was maintaining control of the seizures.

8.8.3 Prescription of Medication

Table 20 summarises the type of professional who prescribed the child's medication. In 92% (n=60) of cases, the children were prescribed medication. In 37% (n=24) of cases, it was a neurologist who prescribed medication. Paediatricians prescribed medication in 31% (n=20) of cases. Other reported professionals included: paediatrician and neurologist (7%; n=3); G.P. (9%; n=6) and "doctor in hospital" (8%; n=5). "Doctor in hospital" could have been either a neurologist or paediatrician, but the parents may have been unsure.

Table 19: Frequency of Seizures

Frequency	N	%
Several a day	7	10.8
1 a day	1	1.5
3-5 a week	3	4.6
1-2 a week	3	4.6
1-2 a month	10	15.4
Less frequent	26	40.0
None now	15	23.1
Total	65	100

Table 20: Professionals Who Prescribed Medication

Prescribing Professional	N	%
Not Prescribed Med.	5	7.7
Neurologist	24	36.9
Paediatrician	20	30.8
Doctor/G.P.	6	9.2
Paediatrician/Neurologist	3	4.6
"Doctor" in hospital	5	7.7
Total	63	97.0

Missing Cases: 2

8.8.4 Age At Which Medication Was Prescribed

The age at which medication started to be prescribed varied from one day old to 18 years of age. Table 21 reports the ages at which medication was prescribed.

Table 21: Age at which Medication was Prescribed

AGE IN YEARS	N	%
1 day old -4 years	20	30.8
5-12 years	20	30.8
13-18 years	18	27.7
Total	58	89.3

Missing Cases: 2

Figure 14 illustrates the percentage of children taking medication. In 86% (n=56) of cases, the children were still taking medication but in 5% (n=3) it had been discontinued. Eight per cent (n=5) of the children had never been prescribed medication. Those who were no longer taking medication were asked to provide information based on past medication.

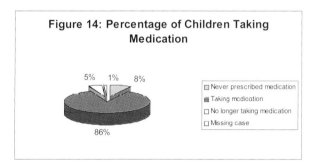

Figure 14: Percentage of Children Taking Medication

- □ Never prescribed medication
- ▦ Taking medication
- □ No longer taking medication
- □ Missing case

In 64% (n=42) of cases, the children's medication was changed a number of times. Twenty eight per cent (n=18) of the children's medication was never changed and 8% (n=5) were never prescribed medication. In two cases, the child was prescribed nine different types of medication over a period of three years. Reasons for alteration or increase in medication included: tiredness, better control of seizures or hand tremors.

Parents' Comments on Changes in Medication

- Changed from Epilim (Sodium Valproate) to Lamictal (Lamotrigine) because Epilim caused hand tremors. Lamictal dosage has increased to 200mg twice daily.
- He was on a smaller dosage (of Epanutin/Phenytoin) and he needed more to control the seizures.
- Tegretol Retard (Carbamazepine) 200mg in the morning was reduced to 100mg because she was very tired.
- Changed from Epilim (Sodium Valproate) to Tegretol (Carbamazepine). On Epilim, X began to loose her speech.
- Different variations were tried to control seizures over a period of three years. At present the combination of Tegretol Retard, Sabril and Frisium seem to control seizures.
- Her seizures have never been controlled and she has been on almost every medication available.
- Phenobarbitone caused drowsiness.
- She was changed from Zarontin (Ethosuximide) to Lamictal (Lamotrigine) at age 18 because it became ineffective, and then to Neurontin (Gabapentin) because Lamictal gave her a rash. Epilim (Sodium Valproate) has been increased from age six.
- Tegretol (Carbamazepine) increased from 200mg B.D. to 300mg B.D. due to breakthrough absence seizures.

Table 22: Names of Prescribed Medication

Type	N	%
Sodium Valproate	40	61.5
Carbamazepine	27	41.5
Lamotrigine	14	21.5
Phenytoin	11	16.9
Tegretol Retard	10	15.4
Phenobarbitone	9	13.8
Gabapentin	7	10.8
Vigabatrin	6	9.2
Clobazam	5	7.7
Diazepam	5	7.7
Clonazepam	5	7.7
Topamax	3	4.6
Ethosuximide	2	3.1
Primidone	2	3.1
Cogentin	2	3.1
Topirimato	2	3.1
Serenace	1	1.5
Corone	1	1.5
Half Inderal La	1	1.5
Valium	1	1.5

- Tegretol gave body rash.
- Tegretol made him sleepy during the day.
- Huge side effects to Phenobarbitone. Hair loss, bad rash and eczema, fevers (became extremely ill).
- At the start she was on liquid Phenobarbitone, then three years later changed to Epilim and Batone Tegretol Retard, tried Epanutin, Sabril, Lamictal, Neurontin, now on Mysoline and Tegretol.
- Epilim on its own was not controlling seizures.

- He has been changed on numerous occasions due to the uncontrolled epilepsy.
- Tegretol didn't work. Ryvifol had severe side effects. Lamictal didn't work. Is on Topamox but still no control.
- Epilim-weight gain one and a half stone in one year. Tegretol-rash. Epanutin-not keeping the epilepsy under control.
- Absences recurred and dose (Epilim) was increased.
- Very difficult to control. Doctors have experimented with many different medications.
- On Tegretol he had an allergic reaction. Neurotin wasn't strong enough.

8.8.5 Medication Prescribed

Table 22 depicts the medication prescribed. The most commonly prescribed drugs were sodium valproate (61.5%; n=40), carbamazepine (41.5%; n=27), lamotrigine (21.5%; n=14) and phenytoin (17%; n=11).

Table 23 shows that in 57% (n=37) of cases, medication was taken in tablet form. Liquid form accounted for 15% (n=10). Combinations of various forms included: tablet and liquid (8%; n=5); liquid and rectal diazapem (5%; n=3); tablet and rectal diazapem (3%; n=2) and tablet, liquid and rectal diazapem (5%; n=3).

Table 23: Forms of Medication

Form	N	%
Doesn't Apply	5	7.7
Tablet	37	56.9
Liquid	10	15.4
Tablet/Liquid	5	7.7
Liquid/Rectal Diazapem	3	4.6
Tablet/Liquid/Diazapem	3	4.6
Tablet/Rectal Diazapem	2	3.1
Total	65	100

Figure 15 shows the number of times a day medication is taken.

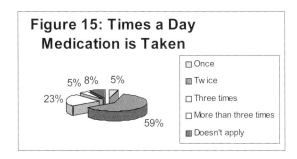

Figure 15: Times a Day Medication is Taken

- □ Once
- ■ Twice
- □ Three times
- □ More than three times
- ■ Doesn't apply

5% 8% 5%
23%
59%

Table 24: Reported Side-Effects of Medication

Side-Effect	Past	Current
Tiredness/Drowsiness	65% (n=42)	31% (n=20)
Lack of Concentration	51% (n=33)	38.5% (n=25)
Memory Difficulties	38.5% (n=25)	29% (n=19)
Headaches	37% (n=24)	11% (n=7)
Moodiness	37% (n=24)	35% (n=23)
Learning Difficulties	34% (n=22)	23% (n=15)
Weight Gain	31% (n=20)	14% (n=9)
Deterioration in sch. wk.	29% (n=19)	21.5% (n=14)
Skin Problems	28% (n=18)	11% (n=7)
Withdrawn	26% (n=17)	17% (n=11)
Dizziness/Visual Disturb.	25% (n=16)	12% (n=8)
Disruptive Behaviour	20% (n=13)	18.5% (n=12)
Gum Swelling	18.5% (n=12)	8% (n=5)
Hyperactivity	17% (n=11)	12% (n=8)
Tantrums	15% (n=10)	14% (n=9)
Nausea/Vomiting	11% (n=7)	1.5% (n=1)
Hormonal Imbalance	9% (n=6)	8% (n=5)
Liver Problems	1.5% (n=1)	0% (n=0)

In 59% (n=39) of cases, the children were reported as taking medication twice a day. Twenty three per cent (n=15) take it three times a day; 5% (n=3) take it four times and 5% (n=3) take it once a day. Eight per cent (n=5) are not taking medication.

8.8.6 Reported Side-Effects of Medication
Table 24 shows the reported side effects that the children on medication have either experienced in the past and/or are currently experiencing. In 74% (n=48) of cases, children are currently experiencing side effects, 18% (n=12) are no longer experiencing side effects and 8% (n=5) are not on medication.

The most notable side effects are education-related: lack of concentration (51%; n=33); difficulties with memory (38.5%; n=25); deterioration in school work (29%; n=19); learning difficulties (34%; n=22). Other side effects which would affect education are tiredness and drowsiness (65%; n=42) and headaches (37%; n=24).

Behavior related side effects were also quite high with 20% (n=13) of parents reporting disruptive behaviour, tantrums (15%; n=10), moodiness (37%; n=24), withdrawn behaviour (26%; n=17) and hyperactivity (17%; n=11).

The reported side-effects of particular drugs are summarised in Table 25.

Table 25: Reported Side-Effects of Particular Drugs

Medication	Side-Effects
Carbamazepine/Tegretol	Headaches, Memory Difficulties, Tiredness/Drowsiness, Gum Swelling, Lack of Concentration, Hallucinations, Nausea/Vomiting, Weight Gain, Skin Problems, Dizziness/Visual Disturbance , Learning Difficulties, Deterioration in School-Work, Disruptive Behaviour, Moodiness, Withdrawn, Hyperactivity, Body Rash
Phenytoin/Epanutin	Nausea/Vomiting, Tiredness/Drowsiness, Gum Swelling, Moodiness, Disruptive Behaviour, Tantrums, Withdrawn
Lamotrigine/Lamictal	Skin Problems Including Hair Growth/Loss, Hormonal Imbalance, Headaches, Dizziness/Visual Disturbance, Skin Rash Lack of Concentration, Moodiness
Sodium Valproate/Epilim	Weight Gain, Hormonal Imbalance, Headaches, Hand Tremors, Nausea/Vomiting, Skin Problems, Tiredness/Drowsiness, Aggression, Disruptive Behaviour, Tantrums, Gum Swelling, Loss of Speech, Hyperactivity, Learning Difficulties, Deterioration in School-Work, Memory Difficulties, Lack of Concentration, Moodiness, Dizziness/Visual Disturbance, Withdrawn, Nose Bleeds
Tegretol Retard	Tiredness/Drowsiness, Lack of Concentration, Headaches, Gum Swelling, Memory Difficulties, Weight Gain, Skin Problems, Hormonal Imbalance
Phenobarbitone	Learning Difficulties, Memory Difficulties, Lack of Concentration, Deterioration in School-Work, Weight Gain, Skin Problems, Hormonal Imbalance, Headaches, Tiredness/Drowsiness, Gum Swelling, Dizziness/Visual Disturbance, Disruptive Behaviour, Tantrums, Moodiness, Withdrawn, Hyperactivity, Skin Rash, Hair loss, Excema
Clobazam/Frisium	Hair Growth, Headaches, Gum Swelling, Dizziness/Visual Disturbance, Learning Difficulties, Memory Difficulties, Lack of Concentration, Withdrawn

Figure 16: Child's Reaction to Taking Medication

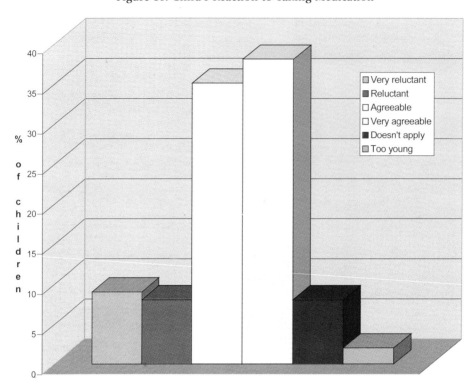

Child's Reaction

8.8.7 Administration of Medication

Table 26 indicates that in 40% (n=26) of cases, the parent administers the medication and in 37% (n=24) of cases the child is responsible for it. In 15% (n=10) of cases both the parent and the child were responsible for the medication, and this was because the children who had to take medication during school were mainly responsible for it themselves.

Table 26: People who Administer the Medication

Person	N	%
Doesn't Apply	5	7.7
Parent	26	40.0
Child	24	36.9
Parent/Child	10	15.4
Total	65	100

Only 28% (n=18) of the children had to take medication in school and they were responsible for it themselves. In only one case, (1.5%; n=1) was medication administered by the school nurse and that was in a special school. All the schools were agreeable to the children taking medication during school hours, but in one case (1.5%; n=1) the parents had not informed the teacher that their child was taking medication in school.

8.8.8 Child's Reaction to Taking Medication

Figure 16 illustrates the child's reaction to taking the anti-epileptic medication. When asked how their children felt about taking medication, 38.5% (n=25) of parents reported that their children were very agreeable and 35% (n=23) were agreeable. Nine per cent (n=6) were reported to be very reluctant while 8% (n=5) were reluctant. One child (1.5%; n=1) was reported to be too young to know.

Figure 17: Frequency of Reassessment

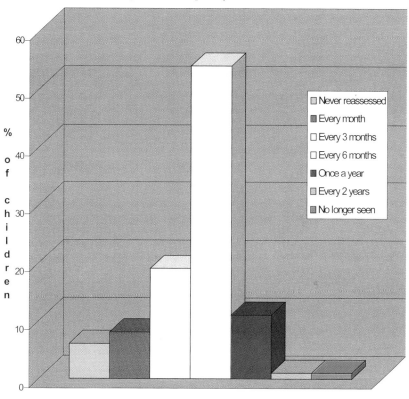

Frequency of Reassessment

8.9   FOLLOW UP ADVISORY AND SUPPORT SERVICES

8.9.1 Frequency of Reassessment

Figure 17 illustrates the frequency of reassessment by specialists. Only 6% (n=4) of parents reported that their children were never re-assessed. The usual period between re-assessment was six months (54%; n=35). In 8% (n=5) of cases, re-assessment was every month and in 18.5% (n=12) of cases, it was every three months. Eleven per cent (n=7) were re-assessed once a year and 1.5% (n=1), every two years. One child is not considered to need re-assessment.

8.9.2 Specialists Conducting Reassessment

In 66% (n=43) of cases, re-assessment was with the same specialist. Six per cent (n=4) were never re-assessed and 28% (n=18) have never seen the same specialist twice. Thirty four per cent (n=22) have asked for their child to be seen by another specialist.

Parents' Reasons for Seeking Another Specialist

- I was not happy with the neurologist.
- The first specialist did not believe that the child was experiencing so many side-effects on Tegretol (Carbamazepine), especially the hallucinations.
- I was anxious to see a neurologist but I was told my child's condition was under control and didn't need to go further.

- Our specialist has, on occasions, consulted with other specialists.
- We were not very happy with our child's behaviour.
- The seizures seem to be more frequent and more severe and she is not getting any help.
- Not satisfied with management of behaviour side and reasons for mood swings.
- We asked to change consultants because X left a lot to be desired. She has been with Y and is now between specialists, as she has turned 18.
- Because of his uncontrolled epilepsy.
- No control of seizures.
- I did ask if I should refer my child to a neurologist but the paediatrician deemed it unnecessary since the medication was controlling the seizures.
- Yes, because of the medication problems. They can't get one to suit her.

8.9.3 Parents' Satisfaction With Monitoring
In 29% (n=19) of cases, parents reported that they were not satisfied with the way in which their child's condition has been monitored by the doctor or specialist since the first diagnosis.

Parents' Reasons for Dissatisfaction with Monitoring
- The following are some of the parents' reasons for their dissatisfaction:
- I was not satisfied with the lack of help from our local health clinic.
- It is very hard to get in touch with them.
- I would like three monthly visits to specialist instead of six monthly.
- Increase of medication appears to be their only solution.
- Anxious to get diagnosis of neurologist.
- Have not seen same doctor and I am not happy with things as they are.
- Initially I would have liked more feedback from the doctor and reassurance about the medications and their side effects.
- Since she has grown older and her epilepsy has become more severe there has been no further information given as to her type of epilepsy or how it affects her.
- Reports get lost. Attitude of doctors at clinic not good. Difficult for my daughter to get proper answers.
- We are very much alone with management of seizures.
- Very bad experiences with X.
- Unhappy with Dr. X -Did not explain anything and seizures continued.
- Annoyed when I wasn't told about her stroke. I had to find out by accident.
- I felt there should have been some blood tests taken.
- I feel that on clinic visits everything is rushed and there is little time to relax and discuss what is happening.
- I would prefer if he was still on a specialist appointment list in hospital.
- I am so frustrated with them acting as if it was not a problem and there is no back up service.

8.9.4 Advice Given by Specialists
In 21.5% (n=14) of cases, no advice was given to parents on how to manage their child's condition: "Nobody told us anything", the comment by one parent, highlights the dissatisfaction expressed by many parents. As indicated in Table 27, the main areas in which advice was given were medication (68%; n=44) and management of seizures (43%; n=28). In 32% (n=21) of cases parents were told to give their child medication without getting any advice or information! In 57% (n=37) of cases, parents were given no advice about management of seizures.

Other areas in which advice was given included: behaviour (14%; n=9); emotional conditions (12%; n=8); and school/education (23%; n=15). In one case, (1.5%; n=1) a parent was told to watch for tiredness and stress levels; another (1.5%; n=1) was told not to allow the child to swim, cycle or drive alone and another (1.5%; n=1) was told to ensure the child wore headgear for sport.

Table 28 shows the sources from which parents obtained information. In 26% (n=17) of cases, it was neurologists who advised the parents. The other main sources of advice were doctors (15%; n=10); paediatricians (11%; n=7) and a combination of neurologists and clinical psychologists (8%; n=5). Other reported sources were: nurses (3%; n=2); G.P. and neurologist (3%; n=2); Brainwave, doctors and books (3%; n=2); Brainwave (3%; n=2); special school that child was

Table 27: Areas In Which Advice Was Given

Area	N	%
Medication	44	67.7
Management of Seizures	28	43.1
School/Education	15	23.1
Behaviour	9	13.8
Emotional	8	12.3

Table 28: Sources of Information

Source	N	%
None Given	14	21.5
Neurologist	17	26.2
Doctor/G.P.	10	15.4
Paediatrician	7	10.8
Neurologist/Clinical Psychologist	5	7.7
Nurses	2	3.1
G.P./Neurologist	2	3.1
Brainwave/Doctor/Books	2	3.1
Brainwave	2	3.1
Hospital/Chemist	1	1.5
Psychologist/Social Worker/Nurse/Specialist	1	1.5
Special School	1	1.5
Total	64	98.5

Missing Case:1

attending (1.5%; n=1); hospital and chemist (1.5%; n=1); psychologist, social worker, neurological nurse and specialist (1.5%; n=1). One parent commented that she had to ask the neurologist for this advice herself.

8.9.5 Needs of Parents
The overall findings in relation to the advisory and support services currently available to parents of children with epilepsy were that in 66% (n=43) of cases, parents feel that their needs are not being met by the services currently provided.

Parents' Needs and Sources of Dissatisfaction
The following are some of the needs and the sources of dissatisfaction referred to by parents:
- Straightforward talk and language we can understand.
- I wish someone had told me what to expect or how to cope or what to do. Taking him home from hospital and not knowing where to turn or what to do-at that time I was so afraid that every time he dropped or took a seizure I thought he was never going to come round.
- More awareness on television, radio, video and newspapers.
- Very little advice given.
- Doctors should listen more to parents.
- More people to listen.
- Meeting parents of other children with similar type of epilepsy and behavioural problems.
- I could not come to terms with my child's condition. I did not know how to handle it and I was given no help. I felt I should have got more back-up from the hospital and some help in trying to come to terms with it.
- More long-term effects/advice and diagnosis.
- I would have liked more support and information.
- Further diagnosis from neurologist.
- From an educational aspect, it would help if systems were in place for children with education-related problems.
- I would like to attend Brainwaves meetings but I am unable to because I live 26 miles from Limerick City where the meetings take place.
- More information on just basics of the illness and its management, the drugs and what the long-term outlook for epileptics are i.e. driving, jobs, documentation-insurance etc.
- I think I should have information as to exactly what type of epilepsy she has and what way it affects her.
- I feel doctors are not able to specify exactly what to expect and as a result my confidence level is low.
- Ideally to see the same doctor who knows her history. Her chart was lost on the first visit to clinic and she was frustrated as no one, not even the doctor, knew her history and she had to repeat it all again. She was very upset.
- I feel a doctor should talk to my son who is 18 now and answer all his questions one to one.
- More information on not just the seizure side of things. It is as if no one knows other difficulties we experience i.e., school and emotional help.
- Again I cannot over emphasise the training professionals must be given in dealing with families of young children recently diagnosed.
- Better communication by neurologist and Health Board.
- Feel child could do with extra attention at school and perhaps he needs counselling.
- Doctors to talk to you more.
- We would be happier if our son was going to school. (This child had finished primary school but was awaiting a place in a special school because of education difficulties caused by his epilepsy).
- I got no information of any kind-only what I poked out myself.
- More government funding so as to raise public awareness of epilepsy. This is too important an issue to have to depend on voluntary contributions.
- I think people should be referred for advice to Brainwave-plain talk without medical terms.
- Management of seizures i.e. dealing with them and advice on coping skills for emotional and behavioural problems for the rest of the family.
- Counselling when my daughter was diagnosed as an epileptic. I knew nothing about it-what to do in a seizure, what to expect when she was having a seizure. It was very frightening at the start.

- Better understanding and knowledge of the condition among teachers.
- Back-up information and help services, particularly with behaviour problems. Helpline and support group. Time off from our daughter.
- There should be meeting groups. In hospital there should be more time spent explaining when first diagnosed. Schools have no knowledge of epilepsy.
- There is no counselling whatsoever.
- As we have a medical background (nurse/laboratory technician) we were at an advantage. Basic explaining is not good and follow-up is poor.
- Get help in managing medication, seizures, behaviour, emotional aspects, school/education.

8.10   EDUCATIONAL PROVISION
8.10.1   Level of Schooling Completed
Figure 18 illustrates the level of schooling completed by the children represented in the sample. In 31% (n=20) of cases, the children had finished pre-school and were currently in primary education; 43% (n=28) had completed primary school and were in secondary education; 17% (n=11) had finished secondary level and were either at third level or doing a training course; 3% (n=2) had completed a third level course. Six per cent (n=4) had not yet started school.

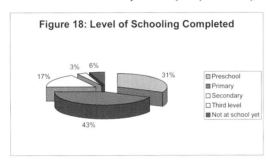

Figure 18: Level of Schooling Completed

In 12% (n=8) of cases, the children were attending either a special school or a special class in a mainstream school. Some of the special schools included Cerebral Palsy Ireland, in Sandymount, St. Paul's Special School, Beaumont, Dublin, St. Declan's, Northumberland Road, Kolbe Centre, Portlaoise, Co. Laois and Catherine Mc Auley Special School, Limerick.

8.10.2   Principals Informed of Child's Condition
When asked if they informed the school principal of their child's condition, 29% (n=19) of parents reported that they had not. In 6% (n=4) of cases the children were not of school-going age. Many parents gave the impression that they were very wary of telling the principal. This might have been the reason so many of them had not informed their children's schools. One parent commented that she had been "dreading telling her and couldn't believe her reaction". Bannon et al. (1992) believes that although epilepsy is a common disorder, it still retains a social stigma that may result in parental reluctance to inform schools. Pond (1981) states that parents are often anxious about rejection arising from the attitudes of others, and these apprehensions range from fear of teasing by other children to fear of rejection by the school.

However, of the 66% (n=43) of parents who did inform the principal, only 6% (n=4) reported that they received an unfavourable reaction. One principal brought someone in to talk to the whole school about epilepsy. Although not an unfavourable reaction, one parent commented that the principal did not know anything about epilepsy and asked her if she could get a booklet on what epilepsy is and what happens to X.

Parents' Comments about Unfavourable Principals' Reactions
- I spoke to the principal before the start of the school year with my daughter present. The reaction was "Oh I hate that. I saw a pupil collapse one day, it was awful". Even though we had explained it was unlikely my daughter would get a seizure, she spoke about my daughter in the past tense: "She <u>was</u> doing so well at school and <u>would</u> have done so well in Leaving Cert.". She spoke as if my daughter was dead.

- Didn't put any emphasis on the condition-could have told him it was sunny outside.
- He wasn't sure my child would be safe.

8.10.3   Class Teachers Informed of Child's Condition
As depicted in Figure 19, 82% (n=53) of parents discussed their child's condition with their child's class teacher(s). Twelve per cent (n=8) reported that they didn't speak with the class teacher and 6% (n=4) of the children had not started school. One parent who had discussed her child's condition with the principal at the time of enrolment was shocked to discover that the principal had not informed the class teacher.

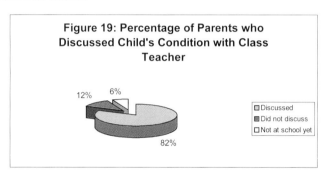

8.10.4   Teachers' Reactions
A higher percentage of parents reported that the class teachers' reactions were more unfavourable than those of the principal. Of the 82% (n=53) of teachers who were informed by parents, 14% (n=9) reacted unfavourably to the news. One parent commented that the teacher informed her she would not know what to do if X had a seizure.

Parents' Comments about Teachers' Reactions
The following are some of the parents' comments about the teachers' reactions when they discussed their child's condition with them:
- Ignorance of epilepsy.
- While admitting to not knowing very much about it, was very understanding and accommodating.
- The answer I got was that nearly every child in the classroom spends a lot of time day dreaming and it would be almost impossible for a teacher to tell the difference between absences and day dreaming.
- They asked what they were to do if she took a fit in school.

In 25% (n=16) of cases, parents thought that teachers were not understanding enough. Even though 57% (n=37) of the parents said their child's teacher was understanding enough, they commented that they felt they were somewhat afraid of the condition and consequently viewed and treated their child differently. The following parent's quote was typical of the general feeling of the parents "I feel they are afraid of the epilepsy and tend to treat X in some ways differently than the other children." One parent reported that some of the teachers attended a lecture on how to deal with it.

Parents' Comments about Teachers' Attitude to their Child's Condition
- They felt I should get them all the information on epilepsy.
- No allowances made with work-load or achievements.
- As my daughter has sub-clinical epileptic activity and shows no real symptoms and still maintains a high standard, I think they find it difficult to understand. As my daughter has said she may be feeling pretty awful, but outwardly looks the same, it is very difficult for a teacher to grasp that she may not be feeling well.
- Because they don't realise the effect on the child with behavioural problems i.e. difficulty with concentration and moods.
- They don't seem to be able to cope with it very well.

- Understanding, after a lot of explaining.
- I'm not sure that they have enough knowledge of the illness.
- They seem to forget that he has epilepsy.
- They don't know enough about it.
- Can't seem to deal with seizures.

8.10.5 Teachers' Knowledge of Epilepsy
When asked if they felt the teacher(s) knew enough about epilepsy, 57% (n=37) of parents reported that they didn't. Only 25% (n=16) of parents thought that the teacher(s) knew enough about the condition. In 12% (n=8) of cases, parents did not inform the teacher(s), so they could not say if the teachers knew enough about the condition. Six per cent (n=4) of the parents were also unable to comment, as their children were not yet at school.

In 45% (n=29) of cases, parents reported that their child was treated the same as other pupils by the teacher. This was sometimes expressed with dissatisfaction because the parents felt that the teacher did not make allowances for their child's condition. In 18.5% (n=12) of cases, parents commented that the teacher had a very appropriate expectation of their child.

In 8% (n=5) of cases, parents reported that their child's teacher accepted work of a lower standard from their child. Eight per cent (n=5) of teachers made less demands of the child; 6% (n=4) had too high an expectation of the child; 5% (n=3) reduced their expectations of the child and 1.5% (n=1) was said to be more lenient about misbehaviour.

8.10.6 Teachers' Awareness of and Contact with Brainwave
Figure 20 illustrates the number of teachers who asked the parents for more information on epilepsy. Forty nine percent (n=32) of teachers asked the parents for more information about their child's type of epilepsy and its management. However, in 33% (n=21) of cases, the teacher(s) did not ask for any information. Twelve per cent (n=8) of teachers were not told about the condition and 6% (n=4) of the children in the sample had not started school.

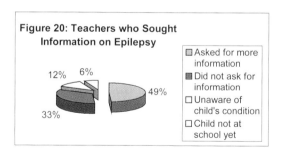

Figure 20: Teachers who Sought Information on Epilepsy

- Asked for more information
- Did not ask for information
- Unaware of child's condition
- Child not at school yet

12%   6%   49%   33%

While parents reported that only 15% (n=10) of the teachers were aware of Brainwave, in 18.5% (n=12) of cases, parents did not know if the teachers were aware of Brainwave because they did not discuss it with them.

Only 8% (n=5) of parents reported that their child's teacher(s) were aware of the support and advisory services that Brainwave offer to schools. In 38.5% (n=25) of cases, the parents did not know if the teachers were aware of these services because they did not discuss it with them.

In 26% (n=17) of cases, parents recommended that the teachers contact Brainwave. However, only 8% (n=5) of parents were convinced that the teacher(s) to whom Brainwave was recommended, had actually contacted Brainwave. In 6% (n=4) of cases, the parents reported that the teachers did not make any contact with Brainwave and in 12% (n=8) of cases the parents did not know if the teachers had made any contact. One parent commented that her child's teacher contacted the hospital neurology nurse and she provided information leaflets for teachers.

8.10.7 Health Board/School Communication

In only 6% (n=4) of cases did the Health Board make contact with the school about the child's condition. Of these, one parent commented that she did not know the reason why the Health Board had contacted her child's school. Another parent reported that contact was made between the Health Board and the school in connection with psychological evaluation and reports regarding remedial help for her daughter. The third parent commented that contact was made regarding domicillary care allowance (this child was attending St. Paul's). The fourth parent did not give any reason for the contact. One parent who came back to Ireland from South Africa commented that in the five years since they returned they have never been contacted by the Health Board regarding their daughter's condition.

8.10.8 Procedures Taken Following a Seizure

Figure 21 illustrates the percentage of teachers who were given guidelines by parents on procedures to take following a seizure.

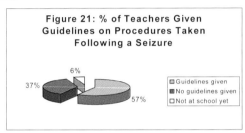

In 57% (n=37) of cases, the parents had given the school precise instructions on what to do if their child had a seizure in school. In 37% (n=24) of cases, teachers had been given no guidelines by the parents. Six per cent (n=4) of children had not been enrolled, so the opportunity for giving instructions had not yet arisen.

Parents' Instructions to Teachers

The following are examples of the type of parental instructions given to teachers:
- Reassure her when she feels dizzy (i.e. seizure commencing). Stay with her, do not try and restrain her. Hold her when the seizure is finished and phone my husband or myself.
- I have a card I received from Brainwave and I will let his teacher have this. It states what to do and how long to leave him before ringing for help.
- Give him plenty of space to help him through the seizure. Afterwards he needs to sleep for about an hour. The school has a room which is suitable for him to rest in. (This child was in secondary school).
- To time the length of the seizure and reassure him if he gets upset-also to inform me.
- Leave her as comfortable as possible. Stay with her. Ring home and 'phone for an ambulance if necessary.
- Reassure him. Ring myself or husband.
- Put child into recovery position and remove any object which he could bang his head on.
- 5mg stesolid and hospital attendance.
- Ensure environment around her is safe. Keep onlookers away. Allow her to move freely-adult to stay with child. When she comes out of seizure allow her to sleep and contact us.
- I told her she must turn X on her side and get an ambulance.
- To place him in a safe place-only if necessary and administer the stesolid. To speak encouragingly to him, reassure him, not to make too much fuss and contact me immediately.
- The school (Catherine McAuley) employs a full time nurse and she is aware of his condition.
- Contact G.P. and parents. Place X in recovery position, loosen all tight clothing and not to administer any medication or drink.
- Loosen tight clothing. Remove any objects that might injure. Place a cushion, pillow or jumper under the head. Place in recovery position.
- Her seizures last 20 to 30 seconds. She is able to continue work afterwards. I have told them to contact me if she hurts herself in a fall, as I work in the school.

- As she is unconscious for such a long time she has to be taken home/hospital. She is turned on her side and I am contacted.
- Phone home. School policy to call ambulance.
- Time seizure. Lie on side. Let the child come round and than call home.
- Not to call an ambulance. Put her into a comfortable position and protect her head. Ring her parents.
- She has a classroom assistant due to uncontrolled seizures.
- Remove the rest of the children from the classroom, leave her on her side and 'phone for me straight away and not to move her at all.

Parent-Reported Procedures that Teachers Employ Following a Seizure
The following are some of the parent-reported procedures that teachers employ when a child is having a seizure in the classroom:
- If there are signs of a seizure beginning they usually try and remove her from the classroom. If she wets herself they change her and follow the above instructions.
- Give 5mg stesolid and attend the nearest hospital.
- Sends the child to the nurse and writes a note in her copy to let us know. (This child was a pupil in Cerebral Palsy Ireland, Sandymount).
- Phone parents to take her home or if after a short rest she seems okay, she stays in school for the rest of the day.
- They move furniture so she does not hurt herself. They make sure she is able to carry on and they inform me of all seizures afterwards.
- They put him to bed as he was in boarding school.
- The first two times they put a spoon in her mouth to hold down her tongue, but now they leave her.

Figure 22 illustrates the frequency of children sent home after a seizure. In 61.5% (n=40) of cases, the parents reported that their child was never sent home from school following a seizure, but in 37% (n=24) of cases, the child had never had a seizure in school so the situation had not arisen. In 23% (n=15) of cases, parents reported that their child was sometimes sent home; 3% (n=2) were often sent home and 6% (n=4) were always sent home. Six per cent (n=4) were not yet at school.

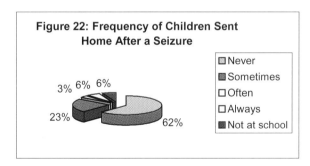

Figure 22: Frequency of Children Sent Home After a Seizure

Legend: Never, Sometimes, Often, Always, Not at school

In 40% (n=26) of cases, the parents agreed with the teachers' decisions in regard to sending their child home, but 6% (n=4) of parents did not agree. In 37% (n=24) of cases, the child never had a seizure in school; 6% (n=4) were not yet at school and 11% (n=7) did not give their opinion regarding the teachers' decisions.

8.10.9 Participation in School-Related Activities
When asked if their child had ever been stopped participating in school-related activities because of their epilepsy, 23% (n=15) reported that they had.

Activities Which Were Restricted
Some of the reported activities and reasons why they were prevented from participating in these included:
- Swimming, in case of drowning.
- Physical Education/Sports and Swimming, at parent's request.

- Physical Education/Sports, Swimming and Work Experience.
- Swimming, because seizures are not fully under control and the pool manager wants letter from doctor to certify that his epilepsy is under control.
- Physical Education/Sports, due to imbalance.
- School Tours-having too many seizures.
- School Tours and Swimming-too much responsibility for teachers.
- Physical Education/Sports and Swimming-too tired.
- Swimming, because parents are not allowed to go with them. Following heated discussion with the person in charge and after a discussion as to why he needs to be supervised, she consented and I was allowed go to supervise him.
- Swimming, afraid it was too dangerous.

According to Thompson and Oxley (1993) restrictions can sometimes adversely influence the development of children with epilepsy and result in underachievement in school and delay in personal development. Holdsworth and Whitmore (1974) reported that head teachers had imposed restrictions on 31% (n=26) of the children with epilepsy attending mainstream schools. However, Tattenborn and Kramer (1992) and Besag (1995) advise that restrictions imposed by teachers and schools should be minimal.

8.11 EDUCATIONAL ACHIEVEMENT
8.11.1 Educational Difficulties
Figure 23 illustrates how the parents felt their child was progressing at school in comparison to their classmates. In 48% (n=31) of cases, parents said that they thought their child was progressing less well than other children their own age. In 34% (n=22) of cases, parents reported that their child was doing as well as other children their own age, while 12% (n=8) of parents felt they were progressing better than children their own age. Six per cent (n=4) were not yet at school.

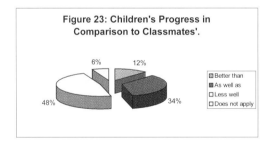

Figure 23: Children's Progress in Comparison to Classmates'.

In 51% (n=33) of cases, parents reported that their child was experiencing educational difficulties. In 43% (n=28) of cases, no educational difficulties were reported by the parents and in 6% (n=4) of cases, the children were not yet at school.

Table 29 shows the reported areas of difficulties experienced by the children. In each area, 6% (n=4) of the sample had not started school. The areas with which the children with epilepsy in this sample had the most difficulties were: concentration (52%; n=34); memory (38.5%; n=25); keeping up in general (35%; n=23); Mathematics (35%; n=23); study skills and routines (31%; n=20) and examinations (31%; n=20). Other areas of reported difficulties were: English comprehension (28%; n=18); English spelling (23%; n=15); English writing (18.5%; n=12); languages (20%; n=13); English reading skills (18.5%; n=12); physical co-ordination (14%; n=9) and speech difficulties (11%; n=7).

In 12% (n=8) of cases the children were either in a special school or a special needs class and in 6% (n=4) they were not yet at school.

Figure 24 illustrates the areas in which remedial help was given. Although 51% (n=33) of children had reported educational difficulties, only 15% (n=10) of the sample were receiving remedial help. Excluding those who were attending special school or in special needs class, 11% (n=7) received help with English, 3% (n=2) with Mathematics and 1.5% (n=1) with Mathematics and English.

Table 29: Areas of Educational Difficulty

Area	N	%
Concentration	34	52.3
Memory Difficulties	25	38.5
Keeping Up In General	23	35.4
Mathematics	23	35.4
Study Skills/Routines	20	30.8
Examinations	20	30.8
English Comprehension	18	27.7
English Spelling	15	23.1
Languages	13	20.0
English Reading Skills	12	18.5
English Writing	12	18.5
Physical Co-Ordination	9	13.8
Speech	7	10.8

Figure 24: Types of Remedial Help

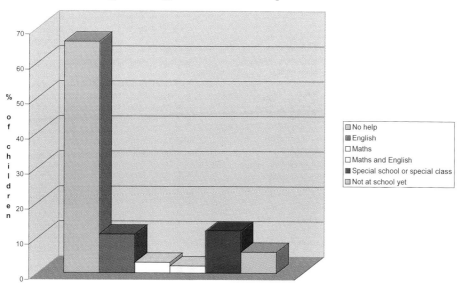

Types of Remedial Help

Legend:
- No help
- English
- Maths
- Maths and English
- Special school or special class
- Not at school yet

In 39% (n=25) of cases, parents reported that they felt their child would benefit from extra educational assistance, either at home or at school. Types of required assistance included: grinds (20%; n=13); remedial help (8%; n=5); help with homework and remedial help (6%; n=4) and help with homework (5%; n=3).

In 54% (n=35) of cases, parents felt that no extra help was required and 6% (n=4) of the children had not yet started school. One parent (1.5%; n=1) did not answer the question.

Parents' Comments about Extra Help
- We would love if there was more support for the subjects she is weak at and some sort of homework club.
- If parents were informed we could help with progress at home.
- Extra tuition early in the morning when she is alert.
- A back-up tuition scheme so she could have a bit more time to understand things that she is hearing.
- Assistance to help X cope with mainstream education difficulties.
- We have home tuition two days a week from the Department of Education this year. Crumlin Hospital helped us arrange this.
- She needs someone to work with her on a one to one basis starting from scratch (Junior Infants level) in Maths.

8.11.2 Effect of Epilepsy on School Progress
When asked if they thought their child's progress at school was significantly affected by their epilepsy, 48% (n=31) of parents reported that they did. In 46% (n=30) of cases, the parents did not feel that their child's condition had affected their progress at school and 6% (n=4) did not comment because their child was not yet at school.

Of the 48% (n=31) whose school progress was reported to have been affected by their epilepsy, 68% (n=21) were affected overall; 19% (n=6) had difficulties with concentration, memory and examinations, 10% (n=3) had Mathematics and language skills difficulties, 3% (n=1) had lack of confidence and difficulties with language skills.

Parents' Comments on the Effects of their Child's Epilepsy on School Progress
- Child had to repeat 4th class because he missed a lot of school due to side effects of medication.
- X is always tired and has a very low concentration.
- She has missed a lot of school and is always struggling to catch up. She also finds it difficult to make friends.
- He loses interest in school work because of his concentration and hyperactivity.
- He was doing very well up to the time of getting epilepsy.
- Concentration, memory, attention span are all very poor. Low self-esteem.
- Goes backward after each seizure.
- I feel that my child was affected by her absence seizures before being put on medication and she lost out on a lot of what was being said by her teacher.
- Since he has gotten epilepsy his standard in school has fallen.
- Pressure of exams and stress bring on seizures. Lack of concentration.
- Difficulty with Maths (poor concentration and memory).
- Poor concentration, reading, taking work down and following instructions.
- He is doing all right in class but at exam time he can't concentrate and his mind goes blank and the teachers were surprised at his results in end of term exams.

When asked if they thought their child's progress at school was significantly affected by the medication they were taking, 46% (n=30) of parents reported that they did. In 3% (n=2) of cases, the children were not at school; 3% (n=2) were neither at school or taking medication and 3% (n=2) were not taking medication.

In 18.5% (n=12) of cases, the parents reported that the medication had an overall negative effect on the children and in 14% (n=9) of cases, the medication made the child very tired and "dopey".

Nine per cent (n=6) of parents reported memory difficulties and tiredness and in one case (1.5%; n=1), the child was said to be aggressive and to display disruptive behaviour.

Parents' Comments on Effects of Medication
- Even though he is not on any medication now, I feel two years on phenobarbitone has affected him.
- She resented the fact she had to take medication and felt her peers were laughing at her.
- Tegretol can have an adverse effect on him and makes him aggressive and abusive at times.
- Lack of memory and tiredness.
- Since he has started medication it has left him relaxed and easy going and his study has suffered.
- She is very tired all the time.
- Reduces her ability and slows down reactions.
- Poor co-ordination, sleepy, sick stomach.
- He seems to be tired a lot of the time and after school he has to go bed as he is stressed out.

8.11.3 Disruptions to Education Attributed to Epilepsy
In 37% (n=24) of cases, parents reported that their child missed out on a lot of school work. In 57% (n=37) of cases, parents reported no difficulties and in 6% (n=4) of cases, the children had not started school.

Reasons for missing a lot of school work included attention and concentration difficulties while in school (12%; n=8); a combination of general absence from school, tonic clonic seizures, attention and concentration difficulties (5%, n=3); general absence from school and attention and concentration difficulties (5%, n=3); general absence from school (3%; n=2); absence seizures while in school (1.5%; n=1); hospitalisation (1.5%; n=1); tiredness and tonic clonic seizures (1.5%; n=1) absence seizures and attention and concentration difficulties (1.5%; n=1)..

Two parents commented that their children are often late for school because of early morning seizures. Another parent said that her child missed a lot of work because she was regularly sent home from school because of behaviour problems.

Table 30 reports the frequency of absences. When asked how many days per month on average, would their child be absent from school because of their epilepsy, 55% (n=36) of parents reported that their child is never absent. In 12% (n=8) of cases, the child is absent one day per month and in 6% (n=4) of cases, they miss four days each month. Other average monthly absences reported included: two days, (5%; n=3); three days (5%; n=3); five days (1.5%; n=1); six days (1.5%; n=1); eight days (1.5%; n=1); nine days (3%; n=2) and ten days (3%; n=2).

Table 30: Frequency of Absences Per Month

Number of Days	N	%
0	36	55.4
1	8	12.3
2	3	4.6
3	3	4.6
4	4	6.2
5	1	1.5
6	1	1.5
8	1	1.5
9	2	3.1
10	2	3.1
Not at School	4	6.2
Total	65	100

One parent reported that his 13 year old daughter attended half of the school year in 1996-1997; one third of the year 1997-1998 and from January to April 1999 she had been in hospital for over a month and now misses three to four days per month.

In 41.5% (n=27) of cases, parents reported that the work or material that their child misses in school is never caught up on. However, 32% (n=21) feel that the work is caught up on and 20% (n=13) said their child doesn't miss out on any work. In 6% (n=4) of cases, the children had not started school.

Parental Comments Regarding Work Missed
- It is not possible to keep up when you miss so much time off school.
- She doesn't catch up on material missed due to failure on her part to get notes etc.
- Most schools don't make allowances for children with epilepsy when they fall behind.
- She can only take in so much at a time and the teachers don't have the time or the patience to go over work she misses.
- Items missed are never gone back over.
- There was no time in the school timetable for catching up.

8.11.4   Department of Education and Science Subject Exemptions and Examination Conditions

Subject exemptions by the Department of Education and Science for children with epilepsy were made in only 5% (n=3) of cases, and in each case it was Irish that was exempted. When asked if they were satisfied with the range of subjects made exempt for children with epilepsy, 74% (n=48) reported that they were unaware of such exemptions. In 25% (n=16) of cases the parents were satisfied, but one parent (1.5%; n=1) was not.

When asked if they were aware that special exam conditions are made available by the Department of Education and Science for children with epilepsy, only 23% (n=15) reported that they were. Only 8% (n=5) of the children in the sample had specific State Examination conditions made available to them when sitting public examinations. In 54% (n=35) of cases such exemptions did not yet apply, as the children were too young.

When asked if they were satisfied with the range of special examination conditions made available to children with epilepsy, 75% (n=49) of parents reported that they were unaware of them, 17% (n=11) said they were happy with them and 8% (n=5) expressed dissatisfaction. One parent commented that she thinks state examinations put too much pressure on a child with epilepsy, and there should be monthly or continuous assessment. Another parent reported that her son did the Leaving Certificate twice and they were never made aware of any special examination conditions.

8.11.5 Aspects of General Development Causing Most Concern

Figure 25 illustrates the aspects of general development which is causing parents most concern.

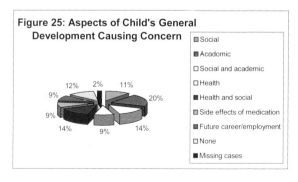

In 20% (n=13) of cases, parents reported that they were most concerned about their child's academic development. Other areas of concern included: social and academic (14%; n=9); health and social (14%; n=9); social (11%; n=7); health (9%; n=6); side effects of medication (9%; n=6);

career and employment prospects (9%; n=6). In 12% (n=8) of cases, the parents had no concerns and in 1.5% (n=1) of cases, no response was received.

One parent commented that she was worried about her daughter, who had become withdrawn because of her condition and was overeating to compensate.

8.12 SOCIAL ADJUSTMENT
8.12.1 Children's Adjustment to Epilepsy
Table 31 summarises how the children felt about having epilepsy. In 12% (n=8) of cases parents reported that they felt that their child was either too young to understand the condition, or had other medical conditions such as Down's Syndrome or Cerebral Palsy, which affected their inhibitions and understanding. In one case, (1.5%; n=1) no response was given to any of the descriptions.

Table 31: Children's Adjustment to Condition

Reaction	N	%
Bothered by it	44	67.7
Regards it as a nuisance	29	44.6
Feels it is unfair	21	32.3
Has a positive attitude	17	26.2
Emotionally upset by it	13	20.0
Uses it as an excuse	9	13.8
Ashamed	9	13.8

In 68% (n=44) of cases, parents reported that their child was bothered by their condition, and in 45% (n=29) of cases they were said to regard it as a nuisance. Thirty two per cent (n=21) of the children felt that it was unfair; 20% (n=13) were emotionally upset by it; 14% (n=9) were ashamed and kept it a secret from their friends; while 14% (n=9) of parents felt that they used it as an excuse. Only 26% (n=17) were reported to have a positive attitude about their condition.

As illustrated in Figure 26, in 59% (n=38) of cases, parents reported that their child had told their classmates that they had epilepsy. However, in 21% (n=14) of cases they had not told their classmates or friends, and 14% (n=9) of the parents did not know whether their child had discussed their condition with their friends. In 6% (n=4) of cases, the children had not started school.

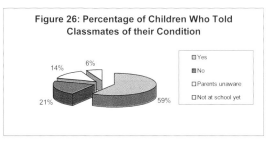

Figure 26: Percentage of Children Who Told Classmates of their Condition

When asked if they felt that their child had fewer friends than other children their own age, 32% (n=21) of parents agreed with this statement. In 8% (n=5) of cases, the parents felt that their child was too young for their condition to have had any affect on their relationships. One parents commented that her child "..has friends but doesn't get to 'play' in their houses as much as other kids".

In 25% (n=16) of cases, parents reported that their children were bullied and teased because of their epilepsy. In 8% (n=5) of cases the parents did not comment because they felt their child was too young.

One parent commented that her daughter felt that her classmates did not understand the problems that she had and because she was "different" the other children didn't get on with her and laughed and called her names.

When asked if their child had difficulty making or keeping friends because of their epilepsy, 18% (n=12) of the parents reported that they did. In 8% (n=5) of cases, the parents felt their child was too young for this to be a problem. One parent commented that her son couldn't keep friends because of his behaviour.

8.12.2   Relationship and Behaviour with Siblings
In 20% (n=13) of cases, the parents reported that their child's epilepsy affected their interaction and relationship with their siblings. However, in 69% (n=45) of cases, parents felt that it had no affect on their relationships, while 11% (n=7) were the only child.

Parents' Comments About Relationships and Behaviour with Siblings
- They are always fighting since she got epilepsy.
- When they are fighting he is jeered about his epilepsy.
- She is angry and difficult to get on with.
- They argue a lot.
- X likes to place herself before others and craves attention.
- She can be aggressive with her sister.
- She tends to feel "put out" and resents her younger sister and brother. She is very immature and resents that they do better at school and have more friends than she had at their age.
- He demands that they do what he wants.
- Her brother finds her behaviour hard to understand.
- Her sister finds it hard to have patience when she has a lot of seizures.
- Her younger sister plays the role of the older sister.
- Can be moody and tired.
- He can pick on one person one day and someone else the next. (There were seven in family).

In 26% (n=17) of cases, parents reported that their child was more badly behaved in the home compared to siblings or other children the same age because of his/her epilepsy.

Parents' Comments About Child's Behaviour in the Home
- Side effects of Epilim is increased aggression. He has gone from being very passive and laid back to very firey and he sometimes gets very physical.
- He is angry a lot since developing epilepsy.
- Very strong minded and this is the cause of arguments and moods.
- He wants his own way all the time.
- She has major behavioural problems.
- Sometimes she thinks she can get away with anything because she's special.

When asked if their child's teacher thought their child was more badly behaved in school because of their epilepsy, 9% (n=6) reported that they did. In 6% (n=4) of cases, the child had not started school.

Parents' Comments about Reported Behaviour At School
- The teacher said that X is becoming very demanding.
- Since developing epilepsy she has had to correct him several times.
- He accuses him of being lazy.
- Doesn't respond well to correction, can be boisterous and disruptive.
- She tended to be very disruptive in class and rarely did homework. The teachers have all noted her behaviour and tend to make allowances because of her epilepsy.
- He plays up on teachers.

Figure 27: Activities Prevented Because of Child's Condition

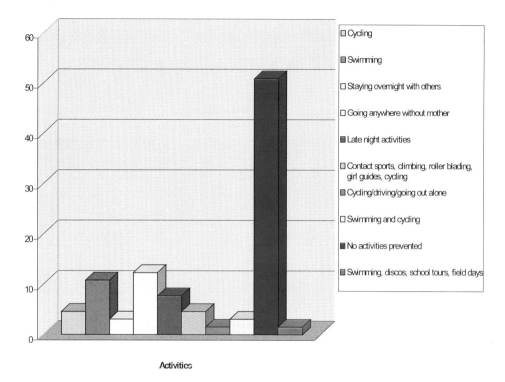

Activities

8.12.3 Limitations on Children's Involvement in Various Activities

In 35% (n=23) of cases, parents reported that their child had fewer interests because of their epilepsy. In 6% (n=4) of cases, parents felt their child was too young for their condition to have affected them yet.

When asked if they limit or prevent any particular activity because of their child's condition, 49% (n=32) of parents reported that they did. Figure 27 illustrates the activities which were prevented. These included: swimming (11%; n=7); late night activities (8%; n=5); cycling (4%; n=3); contact sports, climbing, roller blading, clubs such as Girl Guides or Scouts and cycling (5%; n=3); swimming and cycling (3%; n=2); staying overnight with friends (3%; n=2); cycling, driving and going out alone (1.5%; n=1); swimming, discos, school tours and field days (1.5%; n=1).

In 12% (n=8) of cases, parents reported that they prevented their child from going anywhere without them. This was not restricted to the younger members in the sample.

Parents' Comments about Restrictions

- I just make sure I am with him at all times. I am still afraid to let him go off on any day trips with anyone other than myself or his grandparents.
- Staying overnight with friends if the day has been very active.
- Swimming because of the danger involved.
- I don't like her going to discos because of the lights.
- He wants to go back to swimming lessons but I won't let him until seizures are fully under control.
- When she was younger (12-17) we didn't allow her to go to discos.
- Can't go to junior discos, arcades, etc.

In 54% (n=35) of cases, parents admitted to over-protecting their child because of their epilepsy.

Parents' Reasons for Such Over-Protection

- We feel that she has been through so much during the past six years that we tend to keep her close and in some ways try and protect her from stressful situations.
- I am afraid something might happen him while on his bike or on the stairs or in the bath etc.
- I am frightened because I don't know what is going to happen when I am not around her.
- Because I feel I need to be with her if she ever had a seizure.
- I worry that she might take a seizure and not come out of it.
- I am inclined to make excuses for him and his behaviour.
- Fear of having a seizure when alone.
- I still worry because people expect her to act 19 and I'm afraid people do take advantage.
- He is very innocent and has no sense of danger. It is hard to explain danger unless he experiences it.
- If he has a seizure at school I like him to come home because of embarrassment.
- Always afraid she would take a fit when I would not be around. I worry a lot about her.
- When he goes out at night I have to be up to let him in to know he's all right. He's not allowed to stay over anywhere at night. (20 years of age)

Figure 28 illustrates the activities which parents are reluctant to engage in because of their child's condition. In 20% (n=13) of cases, parents reported that their child's epilepsy made them reluctant to engage in certain family activities. These include: attending public entertainment (12%; n=8); going on family holidays (11%; n=7); visiting friends and relatives (9%; n=6); using public transport (8%; n=5); dining out (6%; n=4) and going shopping (6%; n=4).

Figure 28: Percentage of parents who are Relucatant to Engage their Children in Various Family Activities

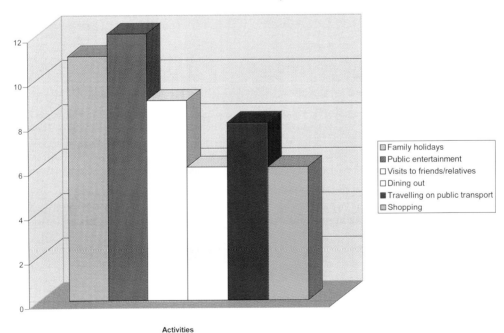

Activities

One parent (1.5%; n=1) did not respond to questions relating to any of the above activities. One parent commented that they couldn't travel on an aeroplane because of her daughter's epilepsy and another parent said they could not go anywhere there was strobe lighting. One family's activities were restricted because "the child has phobias and often wants to go home when we may have just arrived. She get upset for no apparent reason and cries to go home." One parent reported that their child's behaviour can be offputting when the family are going out, but they are learning to deal with it.

8.12.4 Child's Adjustment and General Happiness

Parents reported that in 29% (n=19) of cases, their children have suffered from undue anxiety and depression because of their epilepsy.

Parents' Comments on the General Happiness and Adjustment of their Child with Epilepsy
- Sometimes when she's having a bad bout of seizures she feels very low in herself and wishes she was well.
- When first diagnosed, he was very stressed because the drugs he was on had terrible side effects and the specialist did not believe him. He thought he was going mad. He had to go to Casualty Department twice because of the physical disabilities brought on by stress.
- Anxious about having fits and of knowing whether she has had one or not.
- He is very unsociable.
- Can become sorry for herself and seeks attention and consolation.
- My daughter had great difficulty coming to terms with her epilepsy. We had scenes of anger, frustration and depression. As a family we were patient and sympathetic at first. We tried coaxing but when she started to have self pity we listened for a while but then we changed tactics. We came down heavy on her and told her it was only epilepsy and not cancer or something that would stop her enjoying life to the full. That eventually paid off.
- She gets very depressed because of all the tablets she has to take and the weight she put on. Epilim apparently can cause weight gain and she gets very down because she has a seizure every day. It's a vicious circle.
- Due to strobe lighting she has had to leave discos and plays where they are used. This leaves her feeling a nuisance, as her friends come with her.
- He's just full of stress.
- She is very depressed and anxious. She hears things and sometimes has insomnia. At the onset of a seizure she gets very frightened because of feelings in her legs.
- When she gets up in the morning with the jerking of her limbs and has to cancel the day and go back to bed she gets disappointed.
- He feels his epilepsy is the cause of him having no friends or confidence.

Twenty three per cent (n=15) of the children had attended a psychologist because of behavioural and adjustment problems.

One parent commented that her 19 year old son attended a psychologist because he was bullied in secondary school. Another parent reported that her 18 year old daughter attended a psychologist three times because they discovered that she was in the early stages of anorexia.

Figure 29 illustrates parental reported level of their child's self-confidence. When asked if they felt their child was generally happy and well adjusted, 14% (n=9) of parents reported that they did not. When asked to rate their child's self-confidence, 18.5% (n=12) of parents reported that they were very self-confident; 40% (n=26) were confident; 28% (n=18) were lacking in self-confidence and 12% (n=8) were very lacking in self-confidence. One parent (1.5%; n=1) gave no response.

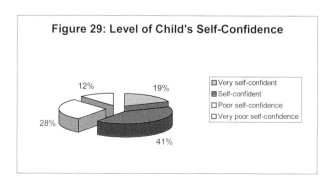

Figure 29: Level of Child's Self-Confidence

125

Figure 30: Areas which Cause Parents Concern Regarding their Children's Future

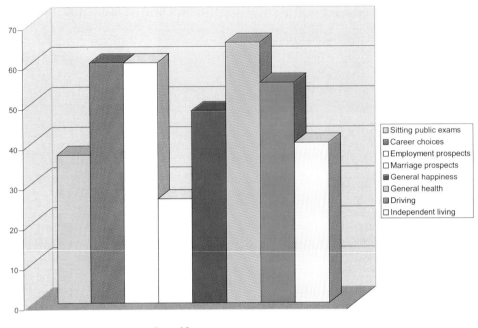

Areas of Concern

Legend:
- Sitting public exams
- Career choices
- Employment prospects
- Marriage prospects
- General happiness
- General health
- Driving
- Independent living

8.13   THE FUTURE

8.13.1 Concerns Regarding the Future

Figure 30 summarises parental areas of concern regarding their child's future. When asked what aspects of their child's future they have concerns about, the following were the most commonly expressed parental concerns: general health (65%; n=42); career choices (60%; n=39); employment prospects (60%; n=39); driving (55%; n=36); general happiness (48%; n=31); independent living (40%; n=26); sitting public examinations (37%; n=24) and marriage prospects (26%; n=17).

For each of the above concerns, 5% (n=3) of parents gave no response. This may have been because their children were very young and they may not have thought about the effect epilepsy may have on their future lives.

When asked if they had any additional concerns other than the aforementioned, 98.5% (n=64) of parents did not express any. One parent (1.5%; n=1) was concerned that her son will be easily influenced and used by other people.

8.13.2 Types of Schools for Children with Epilepsy

When asked to choose which types of school would best provide for their child's specific needs, 62% (n=40) of parents chose mainstream school with special facilities; 6% (n=4) chose special school for children with learning difficulties; 5% (n=3) chose special school for children with emotional disorders and 3% (n=2) chose special school for children with physical handicaps.

The parents were also asked to specify any other type of school which they felt would provide for their child's educational needs. In 31% (n=20) of cases parents stated mainstream education, in 68% (n=44) of cases parents gave no response, and in one case (1.5%; n=1) a parent stated "public secondary school with smaller classes". This child had attended a primary school with small numbers in each class and her parents felt that it would be very difficult for her to cope in a large class in secondary school.

8.13.3 Educational Expectations

Figure 31 illustrates the parents' educational expectations for their children. When asked to state their educational expectations for their child, 60% (n=39) of parents said that they hoped their child would go on to third level; 24% (n=16) hoped they would go on to a training course; 11% (n=7) said they hoped their child would finish second level and 2% (n=1) said they would leave school at 16 years of age. In 3% (n=2) of cases, the parents gave no response.

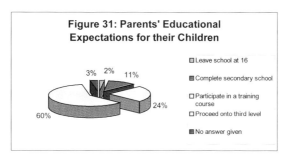

Figure 31: Parents' Educational Expectations for their Children

8.13.4 Parents' Opinions of Irish Educational System

Figure 32 summarises the parents' opinions of the Irish Educational System. When asked to give their views on how the school system has met the needs of their child, parents' opinions indicated a mixture of responses and feelings. In 46% (n=30) of cases, the parents were generally very unhappy about the education system, and the manner in which their child's condition was viewed and treated by the schools. In 31% (n=20) of cases, the parents were generally satisfied; in 6% (n=4) of cases, their child had not started school, so they were unable to comment and in 6% (n=4) of cases the children were in special schools for other conditions and the parents were satisfied with these schools.

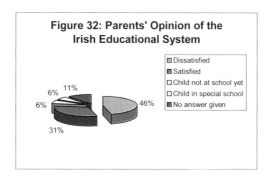

Figure 32: Parents' Opinion of the Irish Educational System

In 11% (n=7) of cases, the parents gave no opinion or felt they could not yet comment, as the following parental comment illustrates: "So far the school has met X's needs (she is in first class). We are at present trying to find a place in a private school, either for children with learning difficulties, or a mainstream school with a special class. As it is early days regarding X's condition, we really would not be in position to comment on how the educational system has met X's educational needs. Perhaps we could tell you in a few years. On a personal note we are delighted this survey is being carried out. Epilepsy is still greatly misunderstood by our generation. Hopefully our children will have a better understanding and not be so afraid of the condition. Explaining our feelings etc. was particularly painful but this survey can only help our little girl and give her the best possible future, which is all we would wish for her. Thank you and good luck."

Positive Parental Comments and Suggestions about the Education System
Positive suggestions
- My daughter is doing well in school but I feel that each school should have a video of what it is like to have a seizure and to show that the child is o.k. afterwards. It would be good for

pupils to learn that it is quite a common condition to have and not to be afraid if they see anyone having a seizure and just to be there when they waken up and keep them as comfortable as possible.

- There should be greater awareness amongst teachers of the possible side effects of epilepsy and associated medication. The school might at least have been in a position to advise of this and recommend some solutions.
- All schools should be furnished with information packs on epilepsy and should make provision for children with this condition i.e. a remedial teacher, a place to lie down and rest following a seizure. Special consideration should be given to people with epilepsy when state exams are being corrected.
- More remedial help is needed in subjects other than English.
- I think training colleges should include medical details of epilepsy and the care of such pupils.
- All teachers should be taught how to deal with a pupil who has epilepsy. All schools should be obliged to have the Epilepsy Association come to the school and advise the students and teachers what happens during a seizure and how to deal with it. The Education Department together with the Health Boards should strive to overcome the stigma associated with epilepsy, especially here in Ireland.
- I think schools should provide behavioural courses and social skills for children with epilepsy because their self awareness and self esteem also seemed to harmed because of their condition.
- We could do with more facilities in schools for people with epilepsy.

Positive experiences
- My son's teacher has been very attentive, kind and loving towards him. I can approach her any time with any worries I may have.
- I found the teacher very helpful with my daughter whenever she took a seizure in class. They would do what they could and always allowed her back to class after.
- The special school has met his needs so far, but it has left him frustrated and with a huge chip on his shoulder. When Rehab was suggested for further training after school, he said "it's for misfits".
- I feel the school has been very supportive. They had previous knowledge of how to react and have never considered excluding her from anything e.g. she was taken to France for two weeks with the school. The only request they made was that I gave the teacher spare tablets in case she lost hers. Teacher never expected her to do anything differently.
- St. Paul's Special School are very well equipped to cater for X's needs. We are very pleased with the school system.
- When she started school four years ago there was no support. After a lot of effort from the school and social worker in Brainwave in Cork we eventually got funding for a classroom assistant and she can now attend school every day. She still gets several seizures every day but she can participate in most things because she has the assistant. It made a huge difference to her life. She has got more confidence now and appears to be a lot happier.

Negative Educational Experiences and Comments Included:
Lack of provision
- I feel that my child is not achieving her full potential since developing epilepsy. She is steadily disimproving and she needs extra attention to improve her concentration skills and self-confidence, but the school cannot offer this "little extra". I feel that she should be given more guidance as regards choice of career because of her condition. Her Junior Cert. results were disappointing and I felt they should be re-examined for signs of "absent spells". I worry a lot about the Leaving Certificate.
- X has attended mainstream school and has reached sixth class. In this time she would have benefited from remedial help but we could not get it. Only two months ago she was assessed by an educational psychologist, after much persuasion, because this is the first year an educational psychologist has been appointed to the area we live. The result of the assessment has shown X to be low average on Mathematics, English comprehension and all learning subjects due to concentration and memory problems.
- X is a bright child who has good comprehension skills. As a result the school totally missed out on the fact that she has learning difficulties. They only saw this when we got her assessed outside. She was four years behind in reading and had major spelling difficulties. The remedial

teacher did not think she needed help and it took us two years to get her into the class. In my view a full time special resource and remedial teacher is required in each school. The teachers do not have the time to give any extra help to an individual child with health problems.

- When I went about looking for a different type of school because X had behavioural problems, I was met with a brick wall from every one down to her old head teacher who said that "whoever came up with the idea of sending her to a special school had not got the child's interest at heart". I was so devastated. I cried for weeks and if it wasn't for the Mater Child Guidance and Dr. X helping us find X Special School I would be almost ill myself as the child suffered terribly from being bullied and made feel stupid for not knowing his tables etc. There is not enough help out there. You have to scream, shout and even cry to get any help in the current education system.

- I feel that there is a lot more that can be done in the area of children with special needs in the school system. Definitely we need more remedial teachers and a programme put in place which will educate teachers to become more aware of children with difficulties at an early stage in the child's education.

- There is no help available in the mainstream schools for children with epilepsy. If you have an obvious physical ailment or mental deficiency you can get assistance, but not with epilepsy as it is not an obvious ailment. In our case, our son did very well in his Junior Certificate, due mainly to the efforts of his mother who spent long hours with him. The school just did not understand or have the knowledge to help him. There is a lack of "education" in the Irish Education System about epilepsy.

Lack of understanding and knowledge of epilepsy

- The school principal and teachers did not know anything about epilepsy. I was quite concerned about X at first because when she first took a small seizure in class her teacher started to shout at her. When the teacher felt she was not concentrating she sent for us and informed us that X was just being bold and would not look at the board when she was teaching. I was very surprised that the teachers in my child's school were unaware of what to do in case of an epileptic fit and questioned should she continue P.E. (This girl was in a special class in secondary school).

- I was surprised with the lack of knowledge at his play school. I think play schools should be included in the education system regarding epilepsy. The schools have been supportive but knew very little about the condition and at times can be anxious and in fear of epilepsy.

- The schools she attended had very dedicated and caring teachers. They did make allowances for my daughter's epilepsy but none of them had any experience with epilepsy and therefore, I don't feel they could really give her the help and understanding that she really needed.

- Her first school was no good as they did not understand her needs. She was bullied there and the teachers would not do anything about it. Even the children's parents treated her like a reject and talked about her in front of their children at home. The second school is better but I'm afraid to tell them about her epilepsy in case she is treated badly again. Teachers need to be made aware of what it is like to have epilepsy. The Irish Education System needs education about epilepsy i.e. understanding of their needs, concentration problems and the need for kindness.

- The career guidance teachers should have more knowledge about epilepsy so they could advise them about suitable occupations.

- It would be nice if teachers had more skills in dealing with epilepsy. Some children have low self-esteem that needs to be developed so that they have the confidence to mix into the mainstream and not go around with a chip on their shoulder. They also need after-school training to help them into the workplace. Children with epilepsy need to be well educated to give them the best quality of life. People in general do not know a lot about epilepsy and they need to be more informed.

- The teachers don't seem to really understand the effects of epilepsy on my son – lack of concentration, poor behaviour, moody, memory problems. I don't think the schools locally are made aware of the special exams conditions. Every secondary school should be made aware of them.

Examinations

- The school was not aware that special exam conditions are available for people with epilepsy. We found that out ourselves and got a letter from her consultant outlining her condition. The

Department of Education replied to this by saying her condition would not be taken into account if she had absentee seizures during exams because, as far as they were concerned it could not be proven. I feel this is an area which should be addressed, as vital points could be lost in five minutes during an exam. This could make a difference to a student's career choice.

- X is currently doing her Leaving Cert. and, today, on the first day of the exam, she suffered a myoclonic jerk seizure. These have been absent for one year so it proves that stress and fatigue are the culprits. Unfortunately, due to the present system, if she suffers a major seizure during the exam she will have to resit her Leaving Cert. next year, when we might have a repeat of the above. I honestly believe that any person who suffers a seizure during an exam should be marked on what was completed.

- We had difficulty with certain teachers in relation to the Leaving Certificate, as they were unaware of specific state examination conditions and this caused frustration for my child. She had partial seizures which caused her to miss first classes over a period of two weeks. I gave a note to her tutor but a certain teacher embarrassed her, even though she explained that her tutor had a note.

- Just to state that my son is suffering at a very bad time, as he is sitting the Leaving Certificate next year and he is finding it extremely hard to catch up and there is no extra support or help available in the school.

- My son is in third level and no allowances were made for failing his exams because of a seizure during one of them. Had to repeat third year. He got 495 points in his Leaving so he has no problems with study.

- I think children with epilepsy should have special concessions in the points system. My daughter will have to go to a private college because she won't be able to get the points needed. If there was an assessment system every few months rather than the Big Exam at the end because it puts too much pressure on the student. My daughter has been put on extra medication because of the pressure of the Leaving Cert.

- I think there is too much pressure on children because of the points system. My child got her first seizure when she was doing the Junior Certificate, but her teachers did not want the bother of looking for special exam conditions when she was doing her Leaving.

8.14 SUMMARY

The responses of the parents were presented in this chapter under headings similar to those used in the questionnaire. In Section 2, biographical details and family circumstances of the children in the sample were documented. Section 3 included information on incidence of epilepsy among family members. Pregnancy and birth circumstances were summarised in Section 4. The developmental history of the children was recorded in Section 5. In Section 6, information on the nature and effectiveness of the children's initial medical referral and diagnosis was compiled. Family reactions to the diagnosis were also examined in this section. Section 7 documented the follow-up advisory and support services which were recommended to parents. Medical issues, such as the children's type and frequency of seizures and their drug-related regimes were compiled in Section 8. Section 9 included information on reassessment and parents' satisfaction with monitoring and the level of support and advice they received. Sections 10 and 11 documented data on the kinds of educational provision to which children with epilepsy had access, and the extent to which such provision met their special educational needs. Information on the educational experiences of the children in the sample and the general level of awareness within the school system of the particular nature and characteristics of children with epilepsy was also presented in Sections 10 and 11. The social adjustment of the children in the sample and the extent to which epilepsy has affected their relationships and social development was documented in Section 12. Parents' concerns and expectations for their children's future, their opinions of the Irish Educational System and the extent to which it has served their children's educational needs were recorded in Section 13.

A full discussion of these findings, and their implications for policy and practice, is outlined in Chapter 9.

CHAPTER NINE
SUMMARY AND RECOMMENDATIONS

9.1 INTRODUCTION

To date, no research whatsoever on the incidence or aetiology of epilepsy among school-going children has been carried out in the Republic of Ireland, and no baseline data on the condition is maintained by any agency of State. The present study reviewed research on epilepsy from the United Kingdom, the United States and Europe in order to establish its relevance to children with epilepsy in Ireland. In particular, the empirical aspects of this study sought to determine the experiences of parents of children with epilepsy and to ascertain their views on the provision currently made available to them in the Republic of Ireland. A sample of parents whose children have epilepsy was selected under the auspices of Brainwave, the Irish Epilepsy Association. These parents were surveyed through a detailed postal questionnaire in order to ascertain their experiences of and views on the medical and educational provision and general service afforded their children by the State.

This chapter reviews the results of the empirical study in light of relevant research findings elsewhere. Educational and medical implications arising from the findings are analysed, and recommendations are made with specific relevance for the Departments of Health and Education and Science. The chapter concludes with a summary statement of the 21 recommendations of greatest significance for the future medical and educational care of children with epilepsy in Ireland.

9.2 BACKGROUND DETAILS

9.2.1 Incidence and Gender of Children with Epilepsy

Of the children surveyed, 6% (n=4) were aged between one and four years; 32% (n=21) were in the four to twelve age group; 35% (n=23) were aged between twelve and eighteen years and 26% (n=17) were aged between eighteen and twenty.

The results of this study further indicated that over half of the sample of children with epilepsy (57%; n=37) were female. This finding contradicts previous studies conducted in this area, but may reflect the fact that this was a volunteer sample.

Studies by Joensen (1986) and Leviton and Cowan (1982) reported a higher incidence of epilepsy among boys. Joensen (1986) also reported that epilepsy seems to be most pronounced in the 5-10 age group of boys. This also contradicts the findings of this study which showed that there was a higher incidence of epilepsy among the girls in the 4-12 age group. These apparently contradictory trends in the data emphasise the urgent need for the compilation and maintenance of an epidemiological database on the incidence and distribution of epilepsy among schoolgoing children in the Republic of Ireland.

9.2.2 Family Circumstances

In 91% (n=59) of cases, the children surveyed were living with both their natural parents. The level of parental separation in this study was very low. This could be due to the fact that the possibility of divorce is a relatively recent phenomenon in Ireland. The National Child Development Study (NCDS) in Britain found that, as a group, one-parent families of children with epilepsy were over-represented, and that divorce and death among such parents were more common than expected (Ross et al. 1980). Betts et al. (1993) also contend that epilepsy can be a focus for conflict in families, resulting in higher rates of separation and divorce in the United Kingdom.

Almost one third (31%; n=20) of the families surveyed in the present study had three children. Twenty six per cent (n=17) had two children and 25% (n=16) had four children. A very low percentage of families (7%; n=5) had more than four children. In 11% (n=7) of cases, there was only one child in the family. The majority of the children sampled (34%; n=22) were the eldest in the family, while 26% (n=17) were in the middle. Although one might presume that the birth of a child with epilepsy could dissuade parents from having further children, the findings of the present study contradict this notion. Only 40% (n=26) of the sample were "only children" or the youngest in their family. The majority (60%; n=39) had younger siblings. However, other factors must be considered when analysing these results. Until comparatively recently, religious prohibitions on birth control held considerable influence in Ireland. Moreover, in the present sample, younger siblings may have been born before the older child was diagnosed as having epilepsy. It is also possible that the parents of the 'only children' or of those who are the youngest in their families may still plan to have more children. These trends in the data can only be confirmed by the regular and recurrent compilation and maintenance of a national database on epilepsy in Ireland.

The results of the present study also showed that an average of 72% (n=46) of parents had completed second level education, 19% (n=12) had completed third level, while 8% (n=5) had completed primary level only. These findings confirm that a considerable majority of the parents sampled had completed second level education only.

9.2.3 Incidence of Epilepsy among Family Members
According to Hauser and Anderson (1986), the children of mothers with epilepsy are more likely to develop epilepsy than are children of fathers with epilepsy. However, the incidence of epilepsy among mothers in this study (8%; n=5) was only marginally greater than the incidence among fathers (5%; n=3). Analysis of the findings further indicated that the incidence of epilepsy within families occurred equally among both paternal and maternal relations. These results contradict findings by O'Connor et al. (1992) who reported that the risk of developing epilepsy appears to be highest when there is previous family history of epilepsy, particularly on the mother's side.

Only 6% (n=4) of the children in the sample had a sibling with epilepsy. It is difficult to comment on the genetic transmission and the incidence of epilepsy among the siblings in this study as, according to O'Donohue (1994), it depends on the type of epilepsy within their family. This is reiterated by O'Connor et al. (1992) who report that in febrile convulsions and petit mal, genetic factors are of paramount importance, but they play a much less significant role in partial epilepsy and in some of the serious epileptic syndromes of infancy and early childhood, e.g., infantile spasms. Such trends in genetic transmission can only be confirmed/disconfirmed by further clinical surveys at national level.

9.2.4 Pregnancy and Birth Circumstances
Complications during pregnancy were reported by 20% (n=13) of the sample. They included: preclampsia, toxemia, gestational diabetes, premature birth, detachment of placenta, removal of gall bladder, near death of mother/baby and other multiple complications. In a Finnish study, Rantakallio and Von Wendt (1986) found prenatal causes in 9% of the children with epilepsy and perinatal causes in 18%.

Birth complications were reported by 40% (n=26) of the present sample. The most frequently reported complications were prolonged labour (25%; n=16) and forceps delivery (19%; n=12). Others included: prolonged delivery, lack of oxygen during birth, caesarian section and mother and baby distressed during birth. In studies from Iceland (Gudmundsson, 1986) and Norway (Krohn, 1961), difficulties during delivery were regarded as constituting the most important aetiological factor.

In 9% (n=6) of cases, the children were diagnosed with epilepsy at birth. Other medical conditions at birth were reported in 14% (n=9) of cases. These included: cerebral palsy, Down's Syndrome, hydrocephalus, asthma, respiratory distress syndrome, congenital adrenal hyperplasia, dislocated shoulder bone and "floppiness at birth". According to Rocca et al. (1987a), epilepsy is significantly more common among persons with cerebral palsy, head trauma and viral encephalits. O'Donohue (1994) also states that seizures may occur in clinical syndromes caused by chromosomal anomalies such as Down's Syndrome. McKusick (1983) comments that there are over 100 single gene disorders which may have epilepsy as a symptom.

The results of the present study therefore indicate that a database on the perinatal complications and medical syndromes associated with epilepsy be compiled by the Department of Health and that such a database be maintained by regular, nationally co-ordinated hospital-based studies of the clinical aetiologies of epilepsy.

9.2.5 Early Developmental History
The most significant developmental problem first identified by parents was in the area of concentration, which 21% (n=14) of parents reported as being non-satisfactory. Other areas of general concern included general alertness (11%; n=7) and behaviour (12%; n=8). However, the majority of parents' comments indicated that the child's development was satisfactory until the first seizure occurred.

9.2.6 Early Symptomatology of Epilepsy
In 3% (n=2) of cases, the parents never suspected that their child had epilepsy. For the other parents, the age at which they suspected their children had epilepsy ranged from one day old to nearly 18 years old. In 38% (n=25) of cases, there were no particular behaviours or warning signs prior to the first seizure. Among the behaviours which caused initial parental concern were twitches, shaking/jerking, trances, febrile convulsions, dizzy spells and unusual head and body movements. These behaviours would indicate that the child had already developed epilepsy but the parents were unaware of it. McGovern (1982) notes in this connection that although seizures occur before the diagnosis, these are usually regarded as 'episodes'; 'something is wrong, but no one is sure what it is.'

9.3   REFERRAL AND DIAGNOSIS PROCEDURES
9.3.1 Early Diagnosis of Epilepsy
In 43% (n=28) of cases, it was the family doctor who carried out the first general medical examination and diagnosed the child as having epilepsy. Other professionals who were reported as having examined the child and made a diagnosis included: paediatricians (37%; n=24), neurologist (14%; n=9) and 'doctors' in the casualty department of the local hospital (6%; n=4). The results of this study indicate that medical personnel occupied differing and sometimes inconsistent roles in the diagnosis of epilepsy, and that this ambivalence and inconsistency caused parents considerable distress.

It is therefore recommended that paediatric departments in hospitals establish a clear diagnostic procedure in cases where epilepsy is suspected in which the roles of the G.P., the paediatrician and the neurologist are clearly defined and their complementary roles in the diagnostic procedure clearly communicated to parents.

In 83% (n=54) of cases, the parents reported that their child attended a neurologist. Although the sample was geographically dispersed across the country, 71% (n=46) of the children attended a neurologist in Dublin. Over half the sample (54%; n=35), reported waiting periods to see a 'public' neurologist that ranged from four to 360 days.

Bearing in mind the emotional trauma associated with the diagnosis of epilepsy, it is further recommended that onward referrals from G.P. to paediatrician or from paediatrician to neurologist should not be unduly delayed, and that where possible a confirmatory diagnosis of epilepsy by a neurologist should be available to parents within one month of the initial referral.

9.3.2 Unambiguous Communication of Diagnosis
The findings of this study suggest that the initial referral and diagnosis procedure caused many parents concern and confusion, both in terms of the manner in which their child's condition was conveyed to them and the lack of information they received. In 26% (n=16) of cases, parents were not told exactly what condition their child had. The term 'epilepsy' was not used in the diagnosis. Instead, euphemisms such as 'episodes', 'attacks', 'seizures', 'fits', or 'turns' were used to describe the child's condition to the parents.

The term used in the diagnosis of the child's condition by the physicians and the ways in which the diagnosis is communicated to parents appear to constitute an essential part of the family's adjustment to the condition. Beech (1992) found that family attitudes, approaches and behaviours towards the child's epilepsy are to some extent shaped by the degree to which family members have an informed understanding of the disorder. Ward and Bower (1978) emphasise that the parents' understanding and acceptance of the diagnosis of epilepsy may depend on the specific terminology used by medical professionals. They found that where the word 'epilepsy' was not used in medical explanations, parents tended to select their own terms and make their own distinctions; for instance, for some a 'convulsion' was not a 'fit' and was therefore less frightening. For others the reverse applied, a 'convulsion' being far worse than a 'fit'. Similarly, some said that 'fits' were not 'epileptic', or not 'really epileptic'; others talked of 'episodes', yet the 'episode' was not a proper 'fit'.

The results of the present study strongly indicate the need for the relevant professionals to communicate the results of a diagnosis of epilepsy unambiguously and sensitively to parents. The word 'epilepsy' should be used immediately after a confirmatory diagnosis is available, and the implications of the condition clearly spelt out in as much detail as is required.

9.3.3 Satisfaction with Information Given

The high level of reported dissatisfaction with the referral and diagnosis procedure (32%; n=21) suggests that the nature and effectiveness of current medical practice urgently needs review. Ambiguous diagnosis, inadequate explanations, lack of information and the use of medical 'jargon' caused much of this dissatisfaction. A number of comments made by parents also indicated dissatisfaction with the cold, clinical manner in which they were informed of their child's condition.

Over one third of the parents (37%; n=24) reported that they were not encouraged to ask questions about the diagnosis, and 41% (n=27) of the parents felt that they were not given enough clear explanations to help them understand and manage their child's condition. Previous studies elsewhere also reported dissatisfaction with both quantity and quality of information provided by medical professionals (Ward and Bower, 1978; Hoare, 1984; Andermann and Andermann, 1992; de Boer, 1995; Tattenborn and Kramer, 1992). According to Andermann (1992), the better educated the person with epilepsy and their carers, the fewer the associated problems. Effective assessment and treatment of epilepsy is dependent upon mutual co-operation and sharing of information between doctors and parents. Parents clearly need to receive more advice and information, not only on medication and management of seizures, but also on the effects of epilepsy on education, behaviour and emotions. Parents also need to be provided with opportunities to ask questions and voice concerns, not only at the time of diagnosis but on a regular and systematic basis thereafter. This concern is incorporated as a Recommendation in Section 9.4.1

9.3.4 Family Reactions to the Diagnosis

McGovern (1992) emphasises that it is a very emotional time for parents when they find out their child has epilepsy. She notes that their reactions to the diagnosis may produce feelings which are similar to those experienced following a bereavement. Reactions expressed by parents in the present study included: anxiety, shock, fear, sadness, confusion, anger, disappointment, guilt, relief, depression, denial and rejection. Analysis of the people whom individual parents told about their child's condition showed that more relations on the mother's side than on the father's side of the family were told. According to McGovern (1982), many fathers look on epilepsy in their child as a slur on their virility, particularly if the child is a son. Wallace (1994) advises genetic counselling for parents, notably those who have a history of epilepsy, as many affected parents, mothers in particular, are likely to feel guilty and may be blamed by their partners for the child's epilepsy.

9.4   FOLLOW-UP SUPPORT AND COUNSELLING SERVICES

9.4.1 Counselling as an Integral Part of the Diagnostic Process

Given that parents' reactions to the diagnosis varied from anxiety to denial and rejection, the importance of counselling and support services cannot be over-emphasised. Yet, 79% (n=51) of the parents in this sample were left to cope with conflicting emotions following the diagnosis without any form of counselling being made available or recommended to them. Parental comments regarding the need for counselling clearly showed that a considerable majority of parents (57%; n=37) needed this support. Parents generally felt that their needs were not being met, and many expressed a wish to have someone to talk to who had experienced similar problems. It is also clear from some parents' comments that they wanted counselling as a means of obtaining more information on epilepsy and its management, as distinct from helping them cope with the situation.

It is therefore recommended that specifically designated and resourced counselling and support services should be made available by the Health Boards as an integral part of the medical diagnosis procedure for the parents of children with epilepsy. The option of genetic counselling should also be made available, and all parents should be informed of Brainwave, the Irish Epilepsy Association and its services at the time of diagnosis.

In 80% (n=52) of cases, parents commented that other support or information would have helped with the particular difficulties which they were experiencing. Parental comments indicated that it would have helped if they could talk to other families in similar situations. This could also be facilitated through a support service organised by the hospital, in association with Brainwave, the Irish Epilepsy Association.

In 20% (n=13) of cases, the parents reported that their child's epilepsy affected their interaction and relationships with their siblings. Many parents commented that siblings found it difficult to understand the condition and that they argued a lot with each other. It has been widely recognised by many researchers that the siblings of the child with epilepsy may also be at risk because of distortions in the family dynamics (Rutter et al., 1971; Hoare, 1984a; Hoare, 1984b; McGovern, 1982; Ferrarri et al., 1983; Hoare and Kerley, 1991). According to McGovern (1992), epilepsy in a child has an inevitable impact on family dynamics. When asked if their child's epilepsy made them reluctant to engage in family activities, 12% (n=8) of parents in the present study reported a reluctance to attend public entertainment, 11% (n=7) were reluctant to go on family holidays, 9% (n=6) were reluctant to visit friends and relatives, 6% (n=4) were reluctant to dine out and 6% (n=4) reported a reluctance to go shopping. These findings would suggest that epilepsy is a condition which affects all family members. Restrictions in family activities may also apply to siblings of the child with epilepsy. There would also appear to be a need for the parallel development of a counselling service for the siblings of children with epilepsy.

It is therefore recommended that the Health Boards should establish central, permanent Regional Assessment Centres in designated hospitals or other appropriate locations throughout the country where information on epilepsy is freely and readily available, where ideas and experiences can be exchanged and to which referrals can be made on an ongoing basis for a multi-disciplinary assessment of children with complicated epilepsy and severe learning difficulties. This facility should be used to secure appropriate educational placement for such children. Regional Assessment Centres should also provide family therapy and other forms of intervention and support for families who may have particular difficulty in accepting or managing the condition.

9.5   MEDICAL ISSUES
9.5.1 Suggested Causes of Epilepsy
In 85% of the cases represented in the present study, there was no cause suggested for the child's epilepsy. According to Sander et al. (1990), no cause is found in the majority of cases of epilepsy (61%). Hauser (1978) states that 65-70% of the cases generally have unknown aetiology, while Chadwick (1990) says that some 70% of epileptic disorders are idiopathic. In this study, the "causes" identified by the medical professionals included: difficult birth circumstances, scar on mesial lobe, insufficient sleep, calcification of the skull, flashing computer screen, 3 in 1 injection, migraine headaches and cerebral palsy.

9.5.2 Types of Epilepsy
In 22% (n=14) of cases, the parents reported that they did not know what type of epilepsy their child had. Although 78% (n=41) of the parents did specify the type, not all were sure that they were correct as many of them added "I think" to their response. This lack of knowledge or uncertainty may be due to the unclear and often ambiguous descriptions they received at the time of diagnosis. As previously shown, 40% (n=26) of parents were confused by the terms used by the doctor or specialist and 37% (n=24) were not encouraged to ask questions about the diagnosis.

9.5.3 Medication

In 92% (n=60) of cases the children were prescribed medication, and in 37% (n=24) of cases the medication was prescribed by a neurologist. Other professionals reported as prescribing medication included: G.P.s, doctors in hospitals and paediatricians. The most commonly prescribed anti-epileptic medications were sodium valproate (62%; n=40); carbamazepine (42%; n=27), lamotrigine (22%; n=14) and pheytoin (17%; n=11). Sodium valproate and carbamazepine have been reported as having fewer side effects than some other medications (Trimble and Thompson, 1984; O'Donohue, 1994). This may explain why they were the most commonly prescribed medications in this study.

In 14% (n=9) of cases, children were prescribed phenobarbitone. This is surprising considering the adverse side effects of this medication. Hutt et al. (1968) found that phenobarbitone had an adverse effect on intellectual tasks involving sustained effort and attention. More recently, Brent et al. (1990) reported that phenobarbitone increased the risk for major depressive illness in children with epilepsy.

In 74% (n=48) of cases, children were reported as currently experiencing side effects of medication. The most notable side effects were education-related. In 46% (n=30) of cases, parents reported that they thought their child's progress at school was significantly affected by the medication they were taking. These included: lack of concentration, memory difficulties, learning difficulties and deterioration in school work. Other reported side effects which would affect education were tiredness and drowsiness and headaches. The frequency of behaviour-related side effects was also quite high, with parents reporting disruptive behaviour (20%; n=13), tantrums (15%; n=10), moodiness (37%; n=24), withdrawn behaviour (26%; n=17) and hyperactivity (17%; n=11). Given these reported side effects, the appropriateness of the continuing use of certain medication is questionable. It would also appear that there is a priority need for regular monitoring of the side effects of the medication as only 8% (n=5) of parents reported that their children are reassessed every month and only 18% (n=12) are reassessed every three months.

It is therefore recommended that the drug regimes of children on medication for epilepsy be regularly reviewed by the Schools' Medical Services at least once a term for schoolgoing children with a view to monitoring, and where necessary changing, drugs or dosages in line with parental and school reports on the child's levels of attentiveness and behaviour.

9.6   EDUCATIONAL CONCERNS

9.6.1 Improved Health Board/School Communication

The Health Board made contact with the school about the child's epilepsy in only 6% (n=4) of cases. The results of the present enquiry indicate an urgent need for improved liaison between medical professionals, the Health Boards and the schools regarding individual children's conditions. An established mechanism for such liaison could also serve to provide teachers with advice regarding appropriate restrictions on school-related activities where such restrictions are necessary. The research evidence from the present study indicates that schools have an important role to play in facilitating the successful adjustment of the child with epilepsy and his/her parents to the condition and to school.

It is therefore recommended that the Schools' Medical Services, in consultation with the proposed Regional Assessment Centres and with the consent of parents, should have direct responsibility for ensuring that principals and class teachers are fully informed as to the nature of the child's condition, so that appropriate attitudes, safeguards and patterns of care are adopted for the child with epilepsy.

Medical professionals should independently advise parents to inform the school about their child's condition. Where necessary, paediatricians and school medical officers should be available to advise the school by means of letter, telephone or visits on the management of the child's condition.

9.6.2 Establishment of a Data Base

A major restriction and limitation on the present study was that at present there is no co-ordinated body of information available in any Governmental Department or Health Board concerning such basic and essential information as the number of children and adults with epilepsy in the State.

A primary recommendation of this study is therefore that the State Department of Health, in conjunction with the Schools' Medical Services and the Health Boards, should compile and maintain a central register of pupils with epilepsy as they progress through the school system so that a consistent record is kept of the management of their condition and that a national database becomes available on children with epilepsy within the education system in the State.

9.6.3 Establishment of In-Service Teacher Training Programmes
Parents' comments about teachers' knowledge and understanding of epilepsy showed that they feel that there is a high level of apprehension among many teachers when dealing with children with epilepsy. In 25% (n=16) of cases, parents thought that teachers were not understanding enough. Although teachers are prepared to admit such pupils to their classes, many parents reported that they tend to treat children with epilepsy differently to other pupils.

It is recommended, in this connection, that the State Departments of Health and Education and Science, Brainwave, the Irish Epilepsy Association and the teacher training institutions should collaborate in designing and providing teacher training modules dealing with the educational, emotional and medical needs of children with epilepsy. This information should be an integral part of existing preservice teacher training programmes, but should also be provided by the Teacher Unions as part of in-service provision for teachers who are already trained. Such programmes should serve to heighten teacher awareness of the possible educational and medical difficulties encountered by many children with epilepsy and the appropriate procedure to follow during and after a seizure. However, such programmes should also be specifically directed towards informing teachers as to how best to maximise instructional and educational opportunities for the child with epilepsy in the classroom.

9.6.4 National Awareness of Epilepsy and Brainwave
The findings of this study suggest that many teachers are unaware of Brainwave, the Irish Epilepsy Association, and the voluntary support and advisory services it offers to schools.

It is therefore recommended that the Departments of Health and Education and Science should combine to financially support Brainwave in their efforts to promote awareness of epilepsy in schools. Such promotion should include a nationwide awareness campaign during a designated week. The follow-up campaign should have an educational focus and should be aimed at teachers, parents and pupils. It should incorporate the development and use of appropriate teaching materials such as videos and information packages located in Teachers' Centres or schools. This annual promotion should help to improve public attitudes towards epilepsy and to reduce the particular problem of the bullying of children with epilepsy in schools.

9.6.5 Extended Psychological Services
A large percentage of the children in the sample were reported to have difficulties with adjusting to their condition. In 68% (n=44) of cases, they were reported to be "bothered by it", 45% (n=29) "regarded it as nuisance", 20% (n=13) were reported to be emotionally upset by their condition and 14% (n=9) were ashamed of it. In 32% (n=21) of cases, parents reported that their child had fewer friends and in 25% (n=16) of cases parents reported that their children were bullied and teased because of their epilepsy. Parents also reported that in 29% (n=19) of cases their children have suffered from undue anxiety and depression because of their epilepsy. It is self-evident that epilepsy is a medical condition with developmental implications which may persist throughout the child's school career and which are often associated with other learning disabilities. It is equally the case that the majority of parents of children with epilepsy in the present study wish their child to be educated in mainstream schools but with appropriate support.

These findings therefore support the urgent need for the extension of the existing school psychological service for children with epilepsy who may have specific cognitive, social and emotional needs. The responsibility of such provision should be met jointly by the Departments of Health and Education and Science.

It is therefore recommended that each Area Educational Psychologist be informed by the Schools' Medical Services or by the proposed Regional Assessment Centres of the number of schoolgoing children with epilepsy in their particular catchment areas, and that the educational psychologist, in consultation with the parents, the school authorities and the special needs teacher, should assume a direct responsibility for monitoring and regularly reviewing such children's educational adjustment and attainment as they progress through primary and secondary school.

9.6.6 Increased Remedial/Compensatory Intervention

Besag (1994) states that, although the details of epidemiological studies show some variability, all of them have reported unequivocally that children with epilepsy are more likely to encounter educational difficulty. Although 51% (n=33) of the children in the sample had educational difficulties, only 15% (n=10) were receiving remedial help. The areas with which the children in this sample had the most difficulties were: concentration (52%; n=34), memory (39%; n=25), keeping up in general (35%; n=23), Mathematics (35%; n=23), study skills and routines (31%; n=20), examinations (31%; n=20), English reading (19%; n=12), comprehension (28%; n=18), spelling (23%; n=15), writing (19%; n=12), languages (20%; n=13) and speech difficulties (11%; n=7). In 11% (n=7) of cases help was provided with English only, and in 3% (n=2) of cases it was provided with Mathematics. However, many parents expressed a wish for the provision of remedial help in other subject areas also.

As a result of educational interruptions such as general absence, hospitalisation, concentration difficulties and absence seizures while in school, many parents commented that they would like individual assistance or home tuition to help their children catch up on material missed. The findings of this study strongly indicate that many children with epilepsy require educational intervention, and that specifically targeted and augmented remedial and resource assistance should be provided.

It is therefore recommended that once a school is notified by the Schools' Medical Services or the proposed Regional Assessment Centres that a particular pupil has epilepsy, the monitoring of this child's educational progress and adjustment at school should become the clear responsibility of the remedial/resource or special needs teacher on the staff. This professional responsibility should transfer and equally apply to the remedial/resource teacher when the child moves from primary to second level school.

In 37% (n=24) of cases, parents reported that their children miss a lot of school work. The reasons for this included a combination of general absence from school, tonic clonic seizures, attention and concentration difficulties, 'absence seizures' while in school, tiredness, and hospitalisation.

It is further recommended that in cases of prolonged or intermittent absence due to illness or hospitalisation, the Department of Education and Science's Home Tuition Scheme should automatically and without undue difficulty be made available for children with epilepsy.

9.6.7 Department of Education and Science Subject Exemptions and Examination Conditions

Another problem facing young people with epilepsy is the issue of subject exemptions and examinations. The only existing official provision made by the Irish Department of Education and Science for students with epilepsy would appear to be in the area of state examinations. Special arrangements exist for candidates with epilepsy who are sitting state examinations. These include:
(1) The provision of a separate room and supervisor if requested by the principal of the school.
(2) If a student has a seizure during an examination, he or she will not be given extra time to finish the paper but will be marked on the part of the paper which has been completed as if it were the full examination. However, in order to qualify for this special consideration candidates must have applied in November of the previous year.

Brainwave, the Irish Epilepsy Association (1991) feel that these arrangements do not cover the full range of difficulties faced by a student with epilepsy. If a person has a seizure before an examination and misses a full paper there is no facility to repeat. There is a strong possibility of a student having a seizure before an examination. It is a stressful time for all pupils but in particular for persons with epilepsy since seizures may be triggered by examination pressure and tension. Students who have partial or 'petit mal' seizures may be refused such concessions because of the difficulty of proving their occurrence. Brainwave, the Irish Epilepsy Association (1998) also comments that not all schools are aware of existing examination concessions and therefore do not apply for them.

Although subject exemptions are made available by the Department of Education and Science under certain conditions of disability or learning difficulty, 74%(n=48) of the parents in the present study were unaware of this. Similarly, only 23% (n=15) of the parents were aware that special examination conditions are available to children with epilepsy when sitting state examinations. However, some parents' comments showed that they have experienced considerable difficulty in obtaining subject exemptions and special examination conditions for their children. These findings suggest that there is an urgent need for increased awareness of such examination conditions and subject exemptions by schools if they are to be in a position to advise parents of their existence. Schools and medical professionals must act as facilitators in this process, as a number of parents reported difficulty in gaining access to such conditions.

It is therefore recommended that Brainwave, the Irish Epilepsy Association, engage in immediate dialogue with the State Department of Education and Science with a view to clarifying the exact conditions under which children with epilepsy may be exempted from taking particular subjects for public examinations, and that the concessionary conditions under which children with epilepsy may take public examinations be unambiguously publicised and made available to parents, the relevant medical professionals and schools.

9.6.8 Career Planning and Vocational Options
Pond (1981) and Thompson and Upton (1992) note that the parents of children with epilepsy express particular concerns regarding their children's future. Results of the survey showed that 60% (n=39) of parents were concerned about career choices and employment prospects for their children. Schools have an important role to play in helping the young person with epilepsy plan for future career choices and employment. It might be appropriate that the Departments of Education and Science and Health should combine to provide funding for Brainwave, the Irish Epilepsy Association and the Irish Association of Career Guidance Teachers to jointly provide career planning initiatives for students with epilepsy.

It is specifically recommended in this connection that career guidance teachers should actively encourage pupils with epilepsy to explore, where appropriate, alternative vocational opportunities such as those provided by the Junior Certificate School Programme (J.C.S.P.), the Leaving Certificate (Applied) Programme and courses provided under the auspices of the National Council for Vocational Awards (N.C.V.A.).

As part of their preparation for dealing with people and attending interviews, the person with epilepsy should be taught how to educate the public about their condition. They need to be taught how to describe their seizures and explain how these affect them and what to do in the event of a seizure. It is essential that children with epilepsy know how to talk about their condition in an informative and factual manner so that no matter what target group is involved, they understand and therefore accept the condition and react appropriately when a seizure occurs.

It is therefore recommended that Brainwave, the Irish Epilepsy Association, should establish a strategic relationship with the Irish Association of Career Guidance Teachers with a view to disseminating advice and information packs on Senior Cycle options, career opportunities, interview techniques and self presentation strategies suited to second-level students with epilepsy.

9.6.9 Educational Provision
When asked to choose which types of schools would best provide for their child's specific needs, 62% (n=40) of parents chose mainstream schools with special facilities; 6% (n=4) chose special schools for children with learning difficulties; 5% (n=3) chose special schools for children with emotional disorders and 3% (n=2) chose special schools for children with physical handicaps.

It is therefore recommended, in accordance with the wishes of the majority of parents of children with epilepsy, that wherever possible, such children be educated in mainstream schools with specially designated facilities for their individual educational needs.

In order to effectively educate children with epilepsy in mainstream schools, the Departments of Education and Science and Health also needs to make the following provisions:

(a) Designation of a Teacher with Medical Needs Training
It is recommended that a designated medical needs teacher be seconded from each school staff for specific training in the management of all medical conditions including epilepsy, and that this teacher be readily available for the management of epileptic seizures and the supervision of the recovery period for children with epilepsy. Such a teacher should be on call for the administration of medication and, in particular, rectal diazapem, where this is deemed necessary.

(b) School Design
In 32% (n=21) of cases, parents reported that their children were sent home following a seizure. However, the results of the present study indicate that it is not always necessary for a child to be sent home following a seizure. After a seizure, sleepiness is a common post-ictal manifestation. According to Besag (1998), all that is often required after such seizures is a short sleep.

It is therefore recommended that in order to facilitate the satisfactory education and integration of pupils with epilepsy in mainstream schools, school planning and design should make specific provision for quiet rooms where children with medical conditions can recover and recuperate before rejoining the class. The availability of such rooms would minimise disruptions to the child's education by allowing the child with epilepsy to remain in school and to return to class when recovered.

9.6.10 Recognition of Epilepsy as a Condition Meriting Particular Educational Provision

Within the present system of education in Ireland, there is an urgent need to recognise epilepsy as a condition warranting some form of supportive education. At present, epilepsy as a condition has no legislative definition, support or recognition in educational provision in the Republic of Ireland. Neither the SERC Report (1993), the publications of the National Council for Curriculum and Assessment nor the recent Education Act (1998) make any reference to epilepsy as a condition requiring special support or provision.

It is therefore recommended that in line with educational legislation in Britain, U.S.A. and most western democracies, the Irish Department of Education and Science specifically includes epilepsy as a medical condition which warrants appropriate educational provision, support and intervention. Such educational provision and intervention would also reflect the legal injunction placed on recognised schools by the Education Act (1998) to "provide education to students which is appropriate to their abilities and needs…and ensure that the educational needs of all students, including those with a disability or other special educational needs, are identified and provided for" [Article 9(a)].

9.7 SUMMARY OF RECOMMENDATIONS

This study has had a public constituency from its inception. It was supported from the outset by Brainwave, the Irish Epilepsy Association. It received a bursary from the Irish National Teachers' Organisation to assist with the empirical aspects of the research. The study is based upon the detailed responses of the parents of children with epilepsy who anxiously await the findings and recommendations of this report in the hope that it will ensure for their children a more equitable recognition of their rights in a democratic society. The 21 recommendations of the study are therefore reiterated in sequence as follows:

1. *That a database on the perinatal complications and medical syndromes associated with epilepsy be compiled by the Department of Health and that such a database be maintained by regular, nationally co-ordinated hospital-based studies of the clinical aetiologies of epilepsy.*

2. *That paediatric departments in hospitals establish a clear diagnostic procedure in cases where epilepsy is suspected in which the roles of the G.P., the paediatrician and the neurologist are clearly defined and their complementary roles in the diagnostic procedure clearly communicated to parents.*

3. *That onward referrals from G.P. to paediatrician or from paediatrician to neurologist should not be unduly delayed, and that where possible a confirmatory diagnosis of epilepsy by a neurologist should be available to parents within one month of the initial referral.*

4. *That the relevant professionals should communicate the results of a diagnosis of epilepsy unambiguously and sensitively to parents. The word 'epilepsy' should be used immediately after a confirmatory diagnosis is available, and the implications of the condition clearly spelt out in as much detail as is required.*

5. *That specifically designated and resourced counselling and support services should be made available by the Health Boards as an integral part of the medical diagnosis procedure for the parents of children with epilepsy. The option of genetic counselling should also be made available, and all parents should be informed of Brainwave, the Irish Epilepsy Association and its services at the time of diagnosis.*

6. *That the Health Boards should establish central, permanent Regional Assessment Centres in designated hospitals or other appropriate locations throughout the country where information on epilepsy is freely and readily available, where ideas and experiences can be exchanged and to which referrals can be made on an ongoing basis for a multi-disciplinary assessment of children with complicated epilepsy and severe learning difficulties. This facility should be used to secure appropriate educational placement for such children. Regional Assessment Centres should also provide family therapy, and other forms of intervention and support for families who may have particular difficulty in accepting or managing the condition.*

7. *That the drug regimes of children on medication for epilepsy be regularly reviewed by the Schools' Medical Services at least once a term for school going children with a view to monitoring, and where necessary changing, drugs or dosages in line with parental and school reports on the child's levels of attentiveness and behaviour.*

8. *That the Schools' Medical Services, in consultation with the proposed Regional Assessment Centres and with the consent of parents, should have direct responsibility for ensuring that principals and class teachers are fully informed as to the nature of the child's condition, so that appropriate attitudes, safeguards and patterns of care are adopted for the child with epilepsy.*

9. *That the State Department of Health, in conjunction with the Schools' Medical Services and the Health Boards, should compile and maintain a central register of pupils with epilepsy as they progress through the school system so that a consistent record is kept of the management of their condition and that a national database becomes available on children with epilepsy within the education system in the State.*

10. *That the State Departments of Health and Education and Science, Brainwave, the Irish Epilepsy Association, and the teacher training institutions should collaborate in designing and providing teacher training modules dealing with the educational, emotional and medical needs of children with epilepsy. This information should be an integral part of existing preservice teacher training programmes, but should also be provided by the Teacher Unions as part of in-service provision for teachers who are already trained. Such programmes should serve to heighten teacher awareness of the possible educational and medical difficulties encountered by many children with epilepsy and the appropriate procedure to follow during and after a seizure. However, such programmes should also be specifically directed towards informing teachers as to how best to maximise instructional and educational opportunities for the child with epilepsy in the classroom.*

11. *That the Departments of Health and Education and Science should combine to financially support Brainwave in their efforts to promote awareness of epilepsy in schools. Such promotion should include a nationwide awareness campaign during a designated week. The follow-up campaign should have an educational focus and should be aimed at teachers, parents and pupils. It should incorporate the development and use of appropriate teaching materials such as videos and information packages located*

in Teachers' Centres or schools. This annual promotion should help to improve public attitudes towards epilepsy and to reduce the particular problem of the bullying of children with epilepsy in schools.

12. That each Area Educational Psychologist be informed by the Schools' Medical Services or by the proposed Regional Assessment Centres of the number of schoolgoing children with epilepsy in their particular catchment areas, and that the educational psychologist, in consultation with the Regional Assessment Centres, the parents, the school authorities and the special needs teacher, should assume a direct responsibility for monitoring and regularly reviewing such children's educational adjustment and attainment as they progress through primary and secondary school.

13. That once a school is notified by the Schools' Medical Services or by the proposed Regional Assessment Centres that a particular pupil has epilepsy, the monitoring of this child's educational progress and adjustment at school should become the clear responsibility of the remedial/resource or special needs teacher on the staff. This professional responsibility should transfer and equally apply to the remedial/resource teacher when the child moves from primary to second level school.

14. That in cases of prolonged or intermittent absence due to illness or hospitalisation, the Department of Education and Science's Home Tuition Scheme should automatically and without undue difficulty be made available for children with epilepsy.

15. That Brainwave, the Irish Epilepsy Association, engage in immediate dialogue with the State Department of Education and Science with a view to clarifying the exact conditions under which children with epilepsy may be exempted from taking particular subjects for public examinations, and that the concessionary conditions under which children with epilepsy may take public examinations be unambiguously publicised and made available to parents, the relevant medical professionals and schools.

16. That Brainwave, the Irish Epilepsy Association, should establishe a strategic relationship with the Irish Association of Career Guidance Teachers with a view to disseminating advice and information packs on Senior Cycle options, career opportunities, interview techniques and self presentation strategies suited to second-level students with epilepsy.

17. That career guidance teachers should actively encourage pupils with epilepsy to explore, where appropriate, alternative vocational opportunities such as those provided by the Junior Certificate School Programme (J.C.S.P.), the Leaving Certificate (Applied) Programme and courses provided under the auspices of the National Council for Vocational Awards (N.C.V.A.).

18. That in accordance with the wishes of the majority of parents of children with epilepsy, that wherever possible such children be educated in mainstream schools with specifically designated facilities for their individual educational needs.

19. That a designated medical needs teacher be seconded from each school staff for specific training in the management of all medical conditions including epilepsy, and that this teacher be readily available for the management of epileptic seizures and the supervision of the recovery period for children with epilepsy. Such a teacher should be on call for the administration of medication and, in particular, rectal diazapem, where this is deemed necessary.

20. That in order to facilitate the satisfactory education and integration of pupils with epilepsy in mainstream schools, school planning and design should make specific provision for quiet rooms where children with medical conditions can recover and recuperate before rejoining the class. The availability of such rooms would minimise disruptions to the child's education by allowing the child with epilepsy to remain in school and to return to class when recovered.

21. That in line with educational legislation in Britain, U.S.A, and most western democracies, the Irish Department of Education and Science specifically includes epilepsy as a medical condition which warrants appropriate educational provision, support and intervention. Such educational provision and intervention would also reflect the legal injunction placed on recognised schools by the Education Act (1998) to "provide education to students which is appropriate to their abilities and needs...and ensure that the educational needs of all students, including those with a disability or other special educational needs, are identified and provided for" [Article 9(a)].

CHAPTER TEN

CONCLUDING PERSPECTIVE

10.1 INTRODUCTION

The purpose of this study was to examine the medical, advisory and educational provision for children with epilepsy in the Republic of Ireland. From the outset, the study received substantial support from Brainwave, the Irish Epilepsy Association. In the absence of any database on the incidence of epilepsy in the Republic of Ireland, the sample of parents of children with epilepsy was selected under the auspices of Brainwave from their database. On account of the central role of Brainwave as the facilitating organisation in the enquiry, and their interest throughout the study, it was deemed appropriate to convey the findings back to this organisation to acquire its perspective on the study. This was done in the form of a structured interview with the Chief Executive of Brainwave, the Irish Epilepsy Association (Appendix 10). The following is a concluding perspective on the interview conducted with the Chief Executive of Brainwave, the Irish Epilepsy Association, in relation to the findings and recommendations of the present study. In particular, the interview sought to establish the general feasibility of the recommendations, the extent to which they applied to Brainwave as the only voluntary organisation for persons with epilepsy in the Republic of Ireland, and their specific relevance to the general improvement of medical and educational provision for children with epilepsy in the Republic of Ireland. This chapter provides an overview of provision for people with epilepsy within the context of the views expressed by the Chief Executive of Brainwave, the Irish Epilepsy Association, and also within the context of the present Irish legislative and constitutional environment.

10.2 ESTABLISHMENT OF A DATABASE

The results of the present study therefore indicate that a database on the perinatal complications and medical syndromes associated with epilepsy should be compiled by the Department of Health and that such a database be maintained by regular, nationally co-ordinated hospital-based studies of the clinical aetiologies of epilepsy.
(Recommendation No.1)

The Chief Executive believes that, although the establishment of a national database is essential, it is highly unlikely, based on Brainwave's previous experience with the Department of Health. All previous attempts to establish a pilot database in a number of the Health Boards have failed. Nonetheless, the findings of the present study confirm the view that this is an extremely urgent issue which Brainwave, the Irish Epilepsy Association, must campaign for. A major restriction and limitation on the present study was that at present there is no co-ordinated body of information available in any Government Department or Health Board concerning such basic and essential information as the number of people with epilepsy. The interview also confirmed the fact that as an organisation, Brainwave does not have sufficient longitudinal data to establish, for example, the exact proportions of people with childhood as opposed to long-term epilepsy. There is also the suggestion that Brainwave's membership may not be representative of different kinds of epilepsy. The establishment of such a database is crucial, if only because the lack of regular, carefully co-ordinated studies of the aetiology and prevalence rate of epilepsy among the Irish adult and child population makes it virtually impossible to establish their medical and educational needs.

According to the White Paper on Early Childhood Education (1999) a National Intellectual Disability Database has been established and planning is already underway to set up a similar database for physical and sensory disabilities. The existence of these databases will assist in planning services and policy at national level. In the absence of accurate statistics for each disability category, only an estimate can be made of the numbers of young children who will require early childhood special education. In the White Paper on Early Childhood Education (1999), it is proposed that each Health Board must also maintain its own database to cover the broad range of disabilities. This collection and recording of data must lead to appropriate planning of intervention services, including early childhood special education, at local level. To do this effectively, it is essential that, within each Health Board, there are well-staffed, multidisciplinary teams available to collate such information and to advise on early intervention strategies recording, planning, development and delivery of services.

10.3 GENETICS AND EPILEPSY
Specifically designated and resourced counselling and support services should be made available by the Health Boards as an integral part of the medical diagnosis procedure for the parents of children with epilepsy. The option of genetic counselling should also be made available, and all parents should be informed of Brainwave, the Irish Epilepsy Association and its services at the time of diagnosis. (Recommendation 5)

The Chief Executive considered that the issue of genetics, in relation to epilepsy, was a particularly valuable aspect of the study. He agreed with the recommendation for genetic counselling, and commented that the genetic aspect of epilepsy is one which is only recently making an impact on workers in the field of epilepsy. He believed that "although many people won't want to hear this, the implications of genetic counselling for prospective parents are considerable." He emphasised the need for counselling services which offer the option of genetic counselling.

However, he expressed surprise at the 66% (n=43) incidence of familial epilepsy and the high percentage of birth complications (40%; n=26). Both were considered to be extremely high. It should be noted here that, according to McMenamin and O'Connor-Bird (1997), some forms of epilepsy, such as absence seizures, generalised tonic-clonic seizures of the idiopathic variety and photosensitive epilepsy have a strong hereditary basis. O'Donohue also (1985) reports that the overall risk to a child of developing epilepsy when one parent has epilepsy is 2%-3%, and where both parents have epilepsy is approximately 25%. It is difficult to comment on the genetic transmission and the incidence of familial epilepsy in the present study as, according to O'Donohue (1994), it depends on the type of epilepsy within the family. As the type of epilepsy the siblings of the children in the present study had was not specified, it is not possible to comment on this aspect of genetic transmission. Such trends in genetic transmission can only be confirmed by further clinical surveys at national level. Again, this emphasises the urgent need for the compilation and maintenance of a database on the clinical aetiologies of epilepsy.

10.4 REFERRAL AND DIAGNOSTIC PROCEDURES
Bearing in mind the emotional trauma associated with the diagnosis of epilepsy, it is recommended that onward referrals from G.P. to paediatrician or from paediatrician to neurologist should not be unduly delayed, and that where possible a confirmatory diagnosis of epilepsy by a neurologist should be available to parents within one month of the initial referral. (Recommendation No. 3)

The Chief Executive believes that early identification of the condition is a critical factor in the family's adjustment to the diagnosis. He also took the view that the recommendation for prompt onward referrals needs to be urgently addressed. The results of this study indicate that not only are diagnoses unduly delayed, but also that medical personnel occupy differing and sometimes inconsistent roles in the diagnosis of epilepsy, and that this ambivalence and inconsistency causes parents considerable distress.

It is recommended that paediatric departments in hospitals establish a clear diagnostic procedure in cases where epilepsy is suspected in which the roles of the G.P., the paediatrician and the neurologist are clearly defined and their complementary roles in the diagnostic procedure clearly communicated to parents. (Recommendation No. 2)

Linked to the issue of early diagnosis is the practice of onward referrals to neurologists for a confirmatory diagnosis. The Chief Executive expressed shock at the large number of children in the present study who were diagnosed by G.P.s. He was very concerned at the high proportions of G.P.s who appear to be making the initial diagnosis, and he believed that the non specialist nature of the preliminary diagnosis of epilepsy is linked to the lack of general information made available to parents about their child's condition. He is of the view that if the diagnosis was coming from the correct source, then parents would receive the information they need and there would not be as much anxiety. According to the Chief Executive, two major contributory factors to the problems encountered in the area of diagnosis are the lack of neurologists in Ireland and the training G.P.s receive in the area of epilepsy.

The acute shortage of neurologists in Ireland is supported by Dr. Houston, Medical Correspondent for the Irish Times (Houston, 2000), who reports that the Mater Hospital has been forced to refuse all new patients with neurological conditions at the out-patient clinic because of a two-year backlog. Dr. Lynch, the only consultant neurologist in the Mater Hospital, also identified a need for a minimum of two outpatient neurological clinics per week, but only one half day is currently available because of space restrictions. He also reported that the beds allocated for neurology patients, which include conditions such as epilepsy, Parkinson's disease and dementia, are constantly occupied by admissions from the accident and emergency unit. According to Dr. Lynch, the Republic of Ireland has one of the worst ratios of consultant neurologists per head of population in Europe. With a population of a similar size, Denmark has 180 neurologists compared to eleven in Ireland (Houston, 2000).

In an article in the Sunday Times Paul Colgan (2001) also reports that waiting times for epilepsy treatments in the Republic of Ireland are expected to double later this year when one of the two neurophysiologists is due to retire. Neurophysiologists provide vital backup to doctors by testing brain and muscle activity. Electroencephalography (EEG) and electromyography (EMG) scans are their main services and are crucial to diagnosing or disproving epilepsy, saving unnecessary surgery. Sean Connolly, the remaining consultant who works as the consultant to three Dublin hospitals, said, "I am working way beyond capacity now, so there is no way I can take on any more work. I have been under increasing pressure as clinicians have become aware of the benefits of neurophysiology, and the requests are coming from all over the country. Demands might increase, but I won't be able to increase my output." He added that if Ireland had the same number of neurophysiologists per head of population as Britain, there would be eleven in the Republic. The Chief Executive of Brainwave commented that neurophysiology was traditionally under-resourced, and a further cutback could seriously delay the diagnosis and treatment of the condition.

The Chief Executive of Brainwave concedes that epilepsy can often be very difficult to diagnose. However, he believes that the fact that G.P.s are trying to diagnose the condition only complicates matters further. He takes the view that if children with suspected epilepsy were referred to a neurologist in the first place there might not be as much anxiety or uncertainty associated with the diagnosis. He is also of the opinion that it is vital that the number of neurologists in the children's hospital services is reviewed nationally, and that the importance of a confirmatory diagnosis by a neurologist is impressed on G.P.s.

The results of the present study strongly indicate that the relevant professionals should communicate the results of a diagnosis of epilepsy unambiguously and sensitively to parents. The word 'epilepsy' should be used immediately after a confirmatory diagnosis is available, and the implications of the condition clearly spelt out in as much detail as is required.
(Recommendation No. 4)

The Chief Executive considers that the unambiguous communication of a diagnosis should be obligatory, not just for epilepsy but for all neurological conditions. The results of the present study confirm that the unambiguous communication of a diagnosis is essential, as the terms used in the diagnosis of the child's condition by physicians and the way in which the diagnosis is communicated to parents constitute an essential part of the family's adjustment to the condition (Ward and Bower, 1978; Beech, 1992). The findings of this survey suggest that the initial referral and diagnosis procedure caused many parents concern and confusion, both in terms of the manner in which their child's condition was conveyed to them and the deficits in the information which they received.

Although previous surveys have also repeatedly emphasised the importance of the communication of the diagnosis of epilepsy, the Chief Executive of Brainwave states that such recommendations have been aimed at the wrong people and should be specifically aimed at physicians, rather than at the Department of Health. He envisages Brainwave as having a role to play in encouraging the medical profession to communicate the diagnosis properly, and he hopes that the Doctor's Pack which was launched by Brainwave in May 2000 will help to address this issue.

10.5 MONITORING OF MEDICATION
It is recommended that the drug regimes of children on medication for epilepsy be regularly reviewed by the Schools' Medical Services at least once a term for school going children with a view to monitoring, and where necessary changing, drugs or dosages in line with parental and school reports on the child's levels of attentiveness and behaviour.
(Recommendation No. 7)

Also linked to the issue of lack of communication on the part of the medical profession is the lack of information concerning medication and in particular its side-effects. The Chief Executive found the attitude of the medical profession to parents' reports of side effects of medication in the present study to be quite significant "..they are just not listening. Parents are telling them, 'Johnny has language problems, Johnny has speech difficulties', but they're not interested. They just want to know how he's reacting to carbamazepine. They are not listening. They're listening to what they want to hear. That is a major problem." Scrambler (1994) reports that failure to consider a patient's view may contribute to non-compliance with treatment for epilepsy. The above recommendation for regular review and monitoring of children's medication, taking account of parental and school reports on the child's levels of attentiveness and behaviour, is essential because effective assessment and treatment of epilepsy is dependent upon a dynamic process of mutual co-operation and sharing of information between the doctor and the patient or the patient's parents, in the case of younger children (The Commission for Control of Epilepsy and it Consequences, 1977; Arangio, 1980; Schneider and Conrad, 1986; Scrambler and Hopkins, 1988; Zeigler, 1981).

10.6 REGIONAL ASSESSMENT CENTRES
It is recommended that the Health Boards should establish central, permanent Regional Assessment Centres in designated hospitals or other appropriate locations throughout the country where information on epilepsy is freely and readily available, where ideas and experiences can be exchanged and to which referrals can be made on an ongoing basis for a multi-disciplinary assessment of children with complicated epilepsy and severe learning difficulties. This facility should be used to secure appropriate educational placement for such children.
(Recommendation No. 6)

The Chief Executive is of the opinion that the recommendation for the establishment of Regional Assessment Centres is of pivotal importance, and is also of extreme urgency as Ireland is the only country in Europe that does not have any kind of epilepsy centre. In the United Kingdom, Belgium and the Netherlands extended mobile outpatient clinics (E.M.O.C.s) which offer specialised treatment and care to people with epilepsy have also been established. De Boer (1995) considers E.M.O.C.s as clearly coinciding with developments in general health care and as being in tune with ethical and economic considerations.

The findings of the present study also suggest that the establishment of Regional Assessment Centres is essential, because close liaison between doctors, neurologists, Health Boards, counsellors, teachers, people with epilepsy and their families is necessary if the child with epilepsy and his or her family are to successfully adjust to the diagnosis and management of the condition. Such centres might provide counselling not only for the child with epilepsy, but also for their siblings and parents, if needed. It is further envisaged that these centres might also cater for other medical conditions such as autism, and for learning disability in general. As an organisation, Brainwave believes that this recommendation applies directly to them in that they have a role to play in the establishment of such centres. Brainwave takes the view that the Department of Health must, as a matter of urgency, establish these Regional Assessment Centres, particularly since the attitudes of governments toward people with epilepsy and their care have been unduly influenced by financial considerations and by ignorance of the precise nature of the condition for far too long.

The proposed Regional Assessment Centres could also serve to facilitate some of the proposals in the White Paper on Early Childhood Education (1999). The White Paper focuses mainly on children from three to six years and covers a wide range of educational needs. It proposes the establishment of an Early Childhood Agency (ECEA) which would ensure a high quality provision of early special education services. It states that parents of all pre-school children with diagnosed disabilities will have access to an early education expert. Initially, the experts' involvement will be as advisers to parents and as disseminators of models of best teaching approaches, and later it may be to teach the children for short periods. Once children with special educational needs begin to attend a pre-school or care facility in which they will receive education, special education advice will be extended to those who work with such children. There will be access to and liaison between specialist advisers, and all teachers will have access to appropriate pre-service and in-service development in relation to this area. The Visiting Teacher or resource teacher will be a significant source of special education support to parents and those who run early childhood facilities. If properly implemented, the proposals contained in the White Paper on Early Childhood Education (1999) are likely to provide much-needed support and have considerable benefits for the health, welfare and education of parents of children with epilepsy, if also for other groups of children with special educational needs.

10.7 PARENTS' SUPPORT GROUPS
Regional Assessment Centres should also provide family therapy and other forms of intervention and support for families who may have particular difficulty in accepting or managing the condition.
(Recommendation No. 6)

The Chief Executive agrees with the need for Parent Support Groups but reports that endeavours to address this issue have been hampered by lack of resources and trained leaders. Past experience has shown that, unless there is a key person to run these groups, they won't survive. He believes that the establishment of rural-based support groups is the most urgent priority, as people in such areas may not have as much access to resources and information about the condition as those living in urban areas. Such groups should cater not only for the needs of parents of children with epilepsy, but also for adults with epilepsy, as a lot of services are directed at children only. Linked to this issue is the development of a web-site by Brainwave to address parents' requests for information about the condition.

However, the results of the present study suggest that although Brainwave, the Irish Epilepsy Association, has made major contributions in providing support to parents of children with epilepsy, a renewed effort, in conjunction with the Department of Health, to establish Parents' Support Groups is critical. In the present study, 80% (n=52) of parents commented that additional support and information would have helped them with the particular difficulties they were experiencing. Given that parents' reactions varied from anxiety to denial and rejection, the importance of counselling and support services cannot be over-emphasised. Parents generally felt that their needs were not being met, and many expressed a wish to talk to someone who had experienced similar problems. It is envisaged that the Regional Assessment Centres, proposed in this and other studies, could also function as venues where parents could meet. Such Parents' Support Groups could provide education and information for target groups such as parents, relations, doctors, teachers and employers who require different kinds of information about epilepsy.

10.8 EPILEPSY AND THE EDUCATION ACT (1998)
It is recommended that in line with educational legislation in Britain, U.S.A. and most western democracies, the Irish Department of Education and Science specifically includes epilepsy as a medical condition which warrants appropriate educational provision, support and intervention. Such educational provision and intervention would also reflect the legal injunction placed on recognised schools by the Education Act (1998) to "provide education to students which is appropriate to their abilities and needs ... to ensure that the educational needs of all students, including those with a disability or other special educational needs, are identified and provided for" [S9 (a)].
(Recommendation No. 21)

Although the condition epilepsy is not specified in the Education Act (1998), it would come under the term 'disability' which is defined as "a condition or malfunction which results in a person learning differently from a person without the condition or malfunction" or "a condition, illness or disease which affects a person's thought processes, perception of reality, emotions or judgement or which results in disturbed behaviour." [S2.1(d-e)]

Some of the aims and objectives of the Act are:
a) *"to give practical effect to the constitutional rights of children including children who have a disability or who have other special educational needs, as they relate to education;*
b) *to provide that, as far as is practicable, and having regard to the resources available there is made available to people resident in the State a level and quality of education appropriate to meeting the needs and abilities of those people;*
c) *to promote equality of access to and participation in education and to promote the means whereby students may benefit from education;*
d) *to promote effective liaison and consultation between schools and centres for education, patrons, teachers, parents, the communities served by schools, local authorities, health boards, persons or groups of persons who have a special interest in, or experience of, the education of students with special educational needs and the Minister."*   [S6]

Further Ministerial functions of the Act are:
a) *"to provide funding to each recognised school and centre for education and to provide support services to recognised schools, centres for education, students, including students who have a disability or who have other special educational needs, and their parents, as the Minister considers appropriate and in accordance with this Act;*
b) *to monitor and access the economy, efficiency and effectiveness of the education system provided in the State by recognised schools and centres of education;"*   [S7.2(a-b)]

Although the Chief Executive states that legally the Department of Education should be providing appropriate forms of education for children with epilepsy, he feels that his experience would tend to indicate that parents will not use the Education Act (1998) as a means of achieving their constitutional rights. He doesn't envisage the Education Act (1998) as automatically enabling people to achieve things without *"..having to fight for them."* However, he believes that the Education Act (1998) will help Brainwave in pursuing individual cases as *"it gives a bit more authority on paper."*

While the Chief Executive believed that the Education Act (1998) would not be used by parents as a means of achieving their constitutional rights, at the time of the interview a judgement on the Sinnott Case had not been handed down. In October 2000, a High Court award of two hundred and fifty five thousand pounds was awarded to Mr. Jamie Sinnott, a 23 year old man with autism, for breach of his constitutional rights when the Irish High Court found that the State had failed to provide for his basic education. The High Court decision that the State's constitutional obligation to provide free primary education for the severely mentally disabled is based on need, not age, and does not stop at eighteen years of age was a landmark ruling. The judgement is presently under appeal to the Supreme Court, pending clarification. Although this case was not contested on the basis of the Education Act (1998), this ruling set precedents for other kinds of disabilities if the State continues to fail to honour its commitments to provide appropriate education for children with special educational needs. According to Oliver (November, 2000), Education Correspondent in the Irish Times, the Department of Education and Science is currently dealing with 58 legal actions from parents of special needs children. Oliver (2000) reports that this is understood to be the tip of a huge iceberg, and that many other parents who believe their children have been treated inappropriately by the State may be waiting in the wings.

The outcome of the landmark Sinnott Case may now herald a new era, not only for children with autism, but for all children with special educational needs. Following the High Court judgment by Justice Barr, the Taoiseach, Mr. Ahern, said that the Government was very conscious that it was a serious matter and that *"there is no doubt that, over the decades, the State failed to provide the sort of education for children with special needs which they have a right to receive."* The Labour Deputy Leader, Mr. Howlin, said that, as a society *"we have to change our ways to ensure that we do not put barriers in the way of anyone trying to vindicate basic rights"* (Oliver, 2000). The Sinnott Case (2000) has significantly raised public awareness, and an increasing number of people with disabilities now recognise their constitutional right to appropriate forms of education. It would now seem appropriate that Brainwave, the Irish Epilepsy Association should use its Newsletter and other resources to increasingly educate parents on their legal and constitutional entitlements and enhance their powers of advocacy in campaigning for appropriate forms of education for their children.

Within the present system of education in Ireland, there is an urgent need to recognise epilepsy as a specific condition warranting some form of dedicated supportive education. At present, epilepsy as a condition has no legislative definition, support or recognition in educational provision in the Republic of Ireland. Neither the report of the governmental Special Education Review Committee (SERC, 1993), the publications of the National Council for Curriculum and Assessment nor the Education Act (1998) make any reference to epilepsy as a condition requiring any form of special support or provision.

10.9 EDUCATIONAL MONITORING

A primary recommendation of this study is that the State Department of Health, in conjunction with the Schools' Medical Services and the Health Boards, should compile and maintain a central register of pupils with epilepsy as they progress through the school system so that a consistent record is kept of the management of their condition and that a national database becomes available on children with epilepsy within the education system in the State. (Recommendation No. 9)

The Chief Executive stated that he was aware of a number of children with epilepsy who are not attending school because of their condition. Without a central register of children with epilepsy, there cannot be an effective system of educational monitoring of children with epilepsy. The National Educational Psychological Services (NEPS), which will be established as an independent statutory agency under the Education Act (1998), has a role to play in such monitoring. It seems reasonable to argue that, once informed by the proposed Regional Assessment Centres or the Schools' Medical Services, each Area Educational Psychologist should assume a direct responsibility for monitoring and regularly reviewing such children's educational adjustment and attainment as they progress through the school system.

The Education (Welfare) Act (2000) is defined as "An Act to provide for the entitlement of every child in the State to a certain minimum education, and, for that purpose, to provide for the registration of children receiving education in places other than recognised schools, the compulsory attendance of certain children at recognised schools, the establishment of a body, to be known as the National Educational Welfare Board, …the identification of the causes of non-attendance on the part of certain students and the adoption of measures for its prevention." It aims to establish a comprehensive legislative and administrative system for dealing in a proactive and preventative manner with school attendance problems and issues relating to the educational welfare of children generally. It will provide for a comprehensive national system which would ensure that children between six to sixteen years of age will attend school, or that if they do not, that they are identified, and that they receive at least a minimum education in order that the State can discharge its constitutional duty in this regard. All children who are to be educated outside the recognised school system, will henceforth be required to register following an assessment of the capacity of the home, or outside body, to provide minimum standards of education. The Education (Welfare) Act (2000) will have important implications for those children with epilepsy who, for varying reasons, have dropped out of school and are not receiving any formal education.

In a critique of the Education (Welfare) Bill (1999), Glendenning (1999) considers it to be a legislative landmark which has the potential to transform the Irish system of education for the coming century. She believes that the reforms proposed in the Bill are praiseworthy, urgently required and long overdue. If implemented, she believes that there is little doubt that the provisions outlined in this courageous and enlightened Bill would remedy many of the existing deficits in the contemporary provision of Irish education. She believed that because the Bill deals with highly sensitive issues such as home education, parental rights, children's rights and the State's right to monitor the education received by its citizens, it was likely to have a controversial passage through the Oireachtas.

The Early Childhood Education Agency, proposed in the White Paper on Early Childhood Education (1999), should also have a particular role to play in educational monitoring. Its stated function will be to ensure high quality of provision of early special education services. The White Paper also requires that providers of early education:

- should *"have the requisite training to provide a service that is effective and have access to further staff development.*
- *are supported by professionals with particular expertise when such is required and by an Inspectorate which will monitor standards and advise in regard to improvements."* [S7.8]

The White Paper on Early Childhood Education (1999) also requires that multidisciplinary teams, representing professionals in special education and health, will be established or expanded, and they will meet to:
- *"consult with and advise parents of a child with disabilities in regard to best options for the education of their child*
- *make decisions with parents in regard to the form of provision that will be made and the location in which it will happen*
- *draft the outlines of an education plan for each child which can be carried out by those involved in the education of the child with assistance and advice from relevant professional as required."* [S7.8]

The National Educational Psychological Services (NEPS), the proposals within the White Paper on Early Childhood Education (1999) and the Education (Welfare) Act (2000) will have a combined role in addressing the present problems connected with educational monitoring of children with epilepsy.

10.10 EDUCATIONAL PROVISION
It is recommended, in accordance with the wishes of the majority of parents of children with epilepsy, that wherever possible such children be educated in mainstream schools with specifically designated facilities for their individual educational needs.
(Recommendation No. 18)

The Education Act (1998) seeks to promote the rights of parents to send their child to a school of their choice and one of its stated objectives is "to promote the right of parents to send their children to a school of the parents' choice" [S6(e)]. As an organisation, Brainwave, the Irish Epilepsy Association, does not support the practice of sending children to England to be educated in the Epilepsy Schools (Brainwave, the Irish Epilepsy Association, 1991). Brainwave prefers mainstream education for children with epilepsy, but acknowledges that there is still a role for a special educational facility for children who have complicated epilepsy and severe learning difficulties interacting with other neurological, environmental and psychological problems.

The Chief Executive believes that, compared to other countries, educational provision for children with epilepsy is the one area in which Ireland has definitely fallen behind. He says that the Department of Education and Science are not sufficiently concerned to uphold the rights of children with epilepsy, and he referred to lack of provision of carers on public transport as a case in point, as bus drivers will not take children with epilepsy on board without a carer.

The recommendations made following an investigation by the Ombudsman in 1998 into the school transport service offered by the Department of Education and Science to a child with spine bifida may also be applied to the issue of school transport for children with epilepsy. The four recommendations were that:
1) Compensation, calculated on the basis of the cost of a daily taxi service to the school, be paid for the hardship caused;
2) The Department of Education and Science devise and publish a school transport scheme for children with special needs and this includes details of the transport grants;
3) Cases involving exceptional circumstances should be dealt with on their merits and not by reference to arbitrary financial restrictions;
4) The published school transport system for children with special needs should include:
   (i) a provision that children with special needs will not, as far as possible,   be disadvantaged by their distance from schools or by their isolation from other such children;
   (ii) details of the rules by which the schemes, including payment of transport grants, is administered;
   (iii) provision for a right of appeal to an official or authority other than the initial decision-maker;

(iv) guidelines used by the DES in making provision for exceptional cases;
(v) provision that the level of transport grants be related to the actual cost of travel by road;
    (Office of Ombudsman, 1998)

In his Report, the Ombudsman said that the particular child on which the above recommendations were based was penalised because he was the only child with disabilities in his particular area. He stated that the school transport system must address the needs of children with disabilities living in isolated areas or at a distance from the school they need to attend. It was also noted that the child was refused transport because the Department of Education and Science could not arrange it within the expenditure limit of nine pounds a day and that the basis for this figure is unclear. The Report stated that procedures for dealing with cases which exceeded the limit were ill-defined and the fact that the particulars of the transport scheme itself were unpublished was contrary to fair and sound administration and could lead to discrimination and different treatment for children in similar circumstances.

The Equal Status Act (2000) will also have legal implications for rights of access to school transport for children with disabilities. It is defined as *'An act to promote equality and prohibit types of discrimination, harassment and related behaviour in connection with the provision of services, property and other opportunities to which the public generally or a section of the public has access, to provide for investigating and remedying certain discrimination and other unlawful activities."* According to the Act *"service means a service or facility of any nature which is available to the public generally or a section of the public, and, without prejudice to the generality of the foregoing, includes – transport or travel"* [S.2].

The Chief Executive feels that although the Department of Education and Science are aware of the problems associated with epilepsy, they choose to do very little about them, preferring to *"..firefight individual cases, rather than implement a policy."* In his experience, the Department of Education and Science will *"..fund nothing ..and the smaller the group, the less likely they are to receive funding. They've a bad attitude."* When dealing with the Department of Education, the Chief Executive reports that Brainwave tends to be more successful when intervening on behalf of individuals in regard to issues such as examinations and carers for transport on buses, than in achieving changes in general policies: *"..they won't respond to applications on a blanket basis, they just won't listen. They tend to take the view that it's the Department of Health's responsibility and so nothing gets done."*

It is recommended that in cases of prolonged or intermittent absence due to illness or hospitalisation, the Department of Education and Science's Home Tuition Scheme should automatically and without undue difficulty be made available for children with epilepsy.
(Recommendation No. 14)

Although the Chief Executive agreed that *"..being without education is a terrible problem for children with epilepsy because it means their quality of life is so awful"* he also believed that the Home Tuition Scheme is one which Brainwave has to be careful about because of the risk that over-protective parents may use it as an excuse for keeping their child at home. However, he agreed that the Home Tuition Scheme should be available for genuine cases when children cannot attend school.

The results of the present study suggest that problems such as choice of school and access to school transport can only be addressed by the establishment of multidisciplinary Regional Assessment Units which could evaluate the appropriateness of mainstream or special education for children with epilepsy, and which could prevent inappropriate referrals to special schools, as happens under the current practice. Arguably, in such a context, the Regional Assessment Units could ensure that each child has access to the most appropriate form of education, and that the requisite form of education is provided through the Home Tuition Scheme if for geographical reasons, transport is unavailable.

10.11 HEALTH BOARD/SCHOOL COMMUNICATION
It is recommended that the Schools' Medical Services, in consultation with the proposed Regional Assessment Centres and with the consent of parents, should have direct responsibility for ensuring that

principals and class teachers are fully informed as to the nature of the child's condition, so that appropriate attitudes, safeguards and patterns of care are adopted for the child with epilepsy. (Recommendation No. 8)

The Chief Executive considers the recommendation that the Schools' Medical Services of the Health Boards should liaise with the school concerning a child's epilepsy as being very important. The results of the present enquiry implicitly indicate an urgent need for improved liaison between the proposed Regional Assessment Centres, the Health Boards' School Medical Services and the schools themselves regarding individual children's conditions. An established mechanism for such liaison could also serve to provide teachers with advice regarding appropriate restrictions on school-related activities where such restrictions are required. The research evidence from the present study indicates that schools have an important role to play in facilitating the successful adjustment of the child with epilepsy and his/her parents to the condition. It would seem to be essential that Brainwave, the Irish Epilepsy Association and the relevant medical professionals should also independently advise parents to inform the school about their child's condition. Where necessary, paediatricians and school medical officers should be available, under the auspices of the proposed Regional Assessment Centres, to advise the school on the appropriate management of the child's epilepsy.

10.12 LEARNING SUPPORT
It is recommended that once a school is notified by the Schools' Medical Services (or the proposed Regional Assessment Centres) that a particular pupil has epilepsy, the monitoring of this child's educational progress and adjustment at school should become the clear responsibility of the remedial/resource or special needs teacher on the staff. This professional responsibility should transfer and equally apply to the remedial/resource teacher when the child moves from primary to second level school. (Recommendation No. 13)

The Chief Executive believes that lack of effective remedial education is a problem area, especially for children who are frequently absent or who experience 'absences' while in school, as there is no remedial provision to bring them back up to the level of the class. The findings of the present study strongly indicate that many children with epilepsy require educational intervention, and that specifically targeted and augmented remedial and resource assistance should be provided.

It is further recommended that each Area Educational Psychologist be informed by the Schools' Medical Services (or the proposed Regional Assessment Centres) of the number of schoolgoing children with epilepsy in their particular catchment areas, and that the educational psychologist, in consultation with the Regional Assessment Centres, the parents, the school authorities and the special needs teacher, should assume a direct responsibility for monitoring and regularly reviewing such children's educational adjustment and attainment as they progress through primary and secondary school.
(Recommendation No. 12)

Although the Chief Executive did not refer to the School Psychological Service, the author believes that the findings of the present study support the urgent need for the extension of the existing clinical and educational psychological services for children with epilepsy who have specific cognitive, social and emotional needs. The responsibility for such provision should be met jointly by the Departments of Health and Education and Science, and consideration should be given to locating a core team from the National Educational Psychological Services in each of the Regional Assessment Centres.

The Government intends to establish the National Educational Psychological Service (NEPS) as an independent statutory agency under the terms of the Education Act, 1998. A comprehensive system will be established by this agency for identifying and assisting all students with learning difficulties. In relation to students with special needs, the principal role of the psychologist will be to consult teachers and parents, to identify the special needs of the student and to make recommendations for appropriate provision.

It is also envisaged that the proposed extended functions of the Inspectorate will help address this area. Section 13 of the Education Act (1998) makes provision for an enhanced Inspectorate, some members of which will be qualified psychologists or persons holding other expertise including expertise in the education of students with special educational needs. The Act also stipulates that inspectors who are psychologists shall have the following functions:

a) *"in consultation with parents to assess the psychological needs of students in recognised schools and to advise as appropriate those students, their parents and the schools in relation to the educational and psychological development of such students;*

b) *to advise recognised schools on policies and strategies for the education of children with special educational needs;*

c) *to advise the Minister on any matter relating to the psychological needs of students in recognised schools;"*   [S13. 4(a-c)]

Both the results of the present study and the view of the Chief Executive in relation to the lack of effective learning support for children with epilepsy strongly reinforce the urgent need for increased remedial and resource provision and the extension of the existing clinical and educational psychological services. It is envisaged that the establishment of the National Educational Psychological Service (NEPS) as an independent statutory agency and the extended functions of the Inspectorate under the Education Act (1998), together with the current general review of special educational provision for children with special needs, will help address the difficulties encountered by children with epilepsy in the education system.

10.13 SUBJECT EXEMPTIONS AND EXAMINATION CONDITIONS

It is recommended that Brainwave, the Irish Epilepsy Association, engage in immediate dialogue with the State Department of Education and Science with a view to clarifying the exact conditions under which children with epilepsy may be exempted from taking particular subjects for public examinations, and that the concessionary conditions under which children with epilepsy may take public examinations be unambiguously publicised and made available to parents, the relevant medical professionals and schools. (Recommendation No. 15)

Although the Chief Executive did not regard the recommendation concerning examination concessions and subject exemptions as being among the most urgent, he did comment that it is an area that needs improvement. He believes that for children with epilepsy, a system of continuous assessment based on the three years of an examination programme, would be much fairer, as the stress related to examinations can trigger epileptic seizures.

The findings of the present study suggest that there is an urgent need for schools to become aware of the precise examination conditions and subject exemptions available to pupils with special educational needs, particularly if they are to be in a position to advise parents of their existence. Only 23% (n=15) of parents in the present study were aware of the existence of examination conditions, while 74% (n=48) were unaware of subject exemptions. As an organisation, Brainwave, the Irish Epilepsy Association is in an opportune position to inform parents of these conditions through their Newsletter, as well as assisting parents in securing such conditions for their children. It is clear that schools, medical professionals and educational psychologists must also act as facilitators in this process, as a number of parents in the present study reported difficulty in gaining access to such provision.

As a result of the Education Act (1998), the National Council for Curriculum and Assessment (NCCA) is now a statutory body of persons appointed by the Minister to assist him with a range of duties relating to the curriculum for primary and post-primary schools and the assessment procedures employed in schools. The development by the NCCA of curriculum guidelines for mainstream education generally also incorporates a strategy in which curricula for students with special educational needs will be addressed. This strategy will provide an overall structure for curriculum development for students with special educational needs. The White Paper on Early Childhood Education (1999) also acknowledges the necessity for appropriate curriculum guidelines to meet the needs of pupils with disabilities and general learning difficulty. It is further acknowledged that adaptations to the curriculum and access to it through the use of assistive technology will be required.

Although Part VIII (Examinations) of the Education Act (1998) refers to preparation and marking of 'papers or materials', no reference is made to adjusted provision for candidates with disabilities. The Report of the Expert Advisory Group on Certificate Examinations (Department of Education and Science, 2000), which submitted recommendations to the Minister for Education and Science on arrangements for assessment of students with special needs stated that "Special arrangements should not put the integrity, status or reputation of the examination at risk." However, in relation to more significant permitted modifications to examination procedures, the Report comments: "When ...elements ... have been waived, .. or the method of examining has been significantly altered, this should be indicated by the presence of an explanatory note on the candidate's certificate of results." It would appear that if the integrity of the system has been maintained, there should be no need for qualifying notes on certificates. Daly (2000) contends that if the changes made to accommodate children with special educational needs are such as to interfere with the integrity of the examination process, the examination should be classified as a different procedure. At present, within the Department of Education and Science there would appear to be a lack of consensus concerning the examination requirements appropriate to children with special educational needs/disabilities. While there is an obvious concern with maintaining the integrity of the public examination system, there is also the problem of how this integrity may be maintained without undervaluing the achievement of students with special needs.

10.14 NATIONAL AND EDUCATIONAL AWARENESS OF EPILEPSY AND BRAINWAVE
It is recommended that the Departments of Health and Education and Science should combine to financially support Brainwave in their efforts to promote awareness of epilepsy in schools. Such promotion should include a nationwide awareness campaign during a designated week. The follow-up campaign should have an educational focus and should be aimed at teachers, parents and pupils. It should incorporate the development and use of appropriate teaching materials such as videos and information packages located in Teachers' Centres or schools. This annual promotion should help to improve public attitudes towards epilepsy and to reduce the particular problem of the bullying of children with epilepsy in schools.
(Recommendation No. 11)

Although individual Community Officers and the Information Officer/Counsellor from Brainwave, the Irish Epilepsy Association, visit a certain amount of schools, their work is hampered by lack of resources and unsatisfactory time-management on the part of the schools. Brainwave envisages the production of information packs for schools as a preferable method of informing the schools about the condition.

Such initiatives would appear to be essential, as the findings of the study suggest that many teachers are unaware of Brainwave, the Irish Epilepsy Association, and the voluntary support and advisory services it offers.

It is recommended that the State Departments of Health and Education and Science, Brainwave, the Irish Epilepsy Association and the teacher training institutions should collaborate in designing and providing teacher training modules dealing with the educational, emotional and medical needs of children with epilepsy. This information should be an integral part of existing preservice teacher training programmes, but should also be provided by the Teacher Unions as part of in-service provision for teachers who are already trained. Such programmes should serve to heighten teacher awareness of the possible educational and medical difficulties encountered by many children with epilepsy and the appropriate procedure to follow during and after a seizure. However, such programmes should also be specifically directed towards informing teachers as to how best to maximise instructional and educational opportunities for the child with epilepsy in the classroom.
(Recommendation No. 10)

The Chief Executive felt that the recommendations of the study concerning teacher education on epilepsy were vital. In the present study, parents' comments about teachers' knowledge and understanding of epilepsy showed that there was a high level of apprehension among many teachers when dealing with children with epilepsy. Although teachers generally are prepared to admit such pupils to their classes, parents reported that they tend to treat children with epilepsy differently to other pupils. This recommendation concerning teacher education is regarded as a core recommendation of the study because while current education policy appears to encourage access to local schools by children with epilepsy, it does not adequately address the issue of the full inclusion of such children in the academic and social life of a school. At present, there is little evidence of the consistent resource provision necessary to promote such inclusion. Information regarding the educational difficulties experienced by children with epilepsy in mainstream education are clearly apparent in the results of the present study. The factors affecting the educational progress of children with epilepsy should be an integral part of existing teacher training courses. The Department of Education and Science should also provide targeted in-service courses on how to maximise the educational opportunities for children with epilepsy.

In the White Paper on Early Childhood Education (1999) it is proposed that steps will be taken that all teachers have access to appropriate pre-service and in-service development to ensure that they have the expert skills and knowledge to develop the potential of pupils with special needs. The White Paper also states that it will be necessary for teachers of children with special needs to update their skills continually to take account of the rapid growth in knowledge of disabilities and the development of best practice in this regard. It is envisaged that a range of induction courses and post-graduate courses will be made available through colleges of education and education support centres to teachers who work specifically with pupils with special needs.

10.15 SPECIAL MEDICAL NEEDS TEACHER
It is recommended that a designated medical needs teacher be seconded from each school staff for specific training in the management of all medical conditions including epilepsy, and that this teacher be readily available for the management of epileptic seizures and the supervision of the recovery period for children with epilepsy. Such a teacher should be on call for the administration of medication and, in particular, rectal diazapem, where this is deemed necessary.
(Recommendation No. 19)

The Chief Executive is of the opinion that the administration of First Aid to children with epilepsy is regarded as another problem area in education, particularly if rectal diazepam is required. He regarded the recommendation for a special needs teacher who could administer medication and who would have specific training in conditions such as epilepsy as a key recommendation of the study, and one which Brainwave would unequivocally support.

It is recommended that in order to facilitate the satisfactory education and integration of pupils with epilepsy in mainstream schools, school planning and design should make specific provision for quiet rooms where children with medical conditions can recover and recuperate before rejoining the class. The availability of such rooms would minimise disruptions to the child's education by allowing the child with epilepsy to remain in school and to return to class when recovered.
(Recommendation No.20)

Although the Chief Executive did not refer to this recommendation for the provision of a quiet room where children can recover following a seizure, it is nonetheless considered to be a very important aspect of the education of children with epilepsy, as research shows that all that is often required following a seizure is a short sleep (Besag, 1998). In order to provide minimal requirements to effectively educate children with epilepsy in mainstream schools, it would seem that the Departments of Health and Education and Science need to make provisions for the training of medical needs teachers and the provision of quiet rooms where the child can recover before returning to class. The availability of such teachers, in conjunction with quiet rooms, would clearly minimise disruptions to the child's education.

10.16 EMPLOYMENT AND EPILEPSY
It is recommended that Brainwave, the Irish Epilepsy Association, should establish a strategic relationship with the Irish Association of Career Guidance Teachers with a view to disseminating advice and information packs on Senior Cycle options, career opportunities, interview techniques and self presentation strategies suited to second-level students with epilepsy.
(Recommendation No. 16)

On the issue of employment for students with epilepsy, the Chief Executive felt that, although there are cases where people with epilepsy are stigmatised, it is more often a case of the candidate being unsuitable for the job. He is of the opinion that most people in society can get a job, regardless of disabilities. He doesn't agree with the assumption that 80% of people with disabilities are unemployed, and believes that nowadays employers "don't give a hoot about colour, creed or anything else", as long as the employees can do the job.

While the Chief Executive may believe that it is easy for people with disabilities to secure employment, recent evidence runs counter to this opinion. A research report entitled 'Visualising Inclusion', conducted by the Kerry Network of People with Disabilities in Ireland (2000), recently reported that just 23% of disabled people in Co. Kerry are employed, although 80% are "ready, able and willing" to work. The research surveyed 104 disabled people about their experiences in education, training, housing and accommodation, transport and participation in everyday life. The Survey found an unemployment rate of 34% among disabled people compared to 9% among the general population in Kerry. Although 23% of those surveyed were in training, the majority were dissatisfied and felt that they were being excluded from meaningful employment. A third had not attended secondary school, and of those who had, basic literary skills were considered to be the main benefit. Just 16% had experienced some form of third-level education. Many of those surveyed said that the reason they did not pursue their education was because they saw no possibility of further progress to education or work. Browne, Chairperson of the Kerry Network of People with Disabilities in Ireland, commented that their research "confirms what we've always known about the exclusion and marginalisation of disabled people." These findings serve to heighten the urgent need for organisations such as Brainwave, the Irish Epilepsy Association, to establish strategic links with the Irish Association of Career Guidance Teachers with a view to disseminating advice and information packs on career opportunities, interview techniques and self-presentation strategies suited to students with epilepsy.

The Chief Executive agrees that people with epilepsy would benefit from interview preparation, and he supported the recommendation that secondary schools should prepare students with epilepsy for interviews. Brainwave also aims to cover self-presentation strategies in the courses they run for people with epilepsy. He reported that Brainwave are trying to educate employers about epilepsy by targeting larger companies such as INTEL and DELL, and also the Trades Unions, with their Employer's Information Pack.

It is recommended that career guidance teachers should actively encourage pupils with epilepsy to explore, where appropriate, alternative vocational opportunities such as those provided by the Junior Certificate School Programme (J.C.S.P.), the Leaving Certificate (Applied) Programme and courses provided under the auspices of the National Council for Vocational Awards (N.C.V.A.).
(Recommendation No. 17)

According to the European Social Fund Evaluation Report: Early Leavers (1996), approximately 14,500 young persons leave the Irish school system each year without having finished the senior cycle of second level education. The Report concluded that the level of provision available to meet the needs of these young people is inadequate. It stressed the need for a more co-ordinated model to assist those who leave early and/or those who are likely to leave school early. Implying that the Irish system of education contained a considerable degree of class bias, the Report concluded that increased relative levels of expenditure on the third level sector, post Leaving-Certificate Courses and the senior cycle of second level education has meant that the balance of labour market advantage is moving in favour of the relatively more advantaged in Irish society. The Report recommended a concentration of resources on this chronically marginalised group coupled with a radical restructuring of what is now merely "a notional facilitatory framework that purportedly serves to advance them through the system."

The findings of both the Report, 'Visualising Inclusion' (Kerry Network of People with Disabilities in Ireland, 2000) and the European Social Fund Evaluation Report: Early Leavers (1996) confirm that it is essential that students with epilepsy are encouraged to actively explore alternative vocational opportunities such as the Applied and Leaving Certificate Course so that they do not decide to abandon second level education. Under the terms of the Education Act (1998) one of the functions of the school is to "ensure that students have access to appropriate guidance to assist them in their educational and career choices" [S9. (c)]. It is imperative that career guidance teachers are sufficiently informed about epilepsy to enable them to advise students with epilepsy regarding career opportunities or, where appropriate, alternative vocational opportunities.

10.17 THE CURRENT LEGISLATIVE AND CONSTITUTIONAL ENVIRONMENT

Over the past decade, a number of quite significant developments in special needs education have occurred in Ireland, and provision for all such children is increasingly envisaged as forming a continuum. In recent years, there has also been a sequence of developments of great importance for the welfare of children generally. The United Nations Convention on Children's Rights, 1990, ratified by Ireland in 1992, was a historic landmark with regard to societal dispositions towards the welfare of children with special needs. Another landmark was the enactment of Ireland's first comprehensive legislation on children's welfare since independence, the Child Care Act of 1991. This Act places a statutory duty on Health Boards to identify and promote the welfare of children who are not receiving adequate care, and obliges them to provide a range of child care family support. From the 1990s onwards, increased attention has been devoted to special needs issues, as illustrated by the Special Education Review Committee (SERC) Report (1993), the Government White Paper on Education, Charting our Education Future (1996), the Report of the Governmental Commission on the Status of People with Disabilities, A Strategy for Equality (1996), the Education Act (1998) and the NCCA Discussion Document (1999), Special Educational Needs: Curriculum Issues and the National Children's Strategy (2000).

It is hoped that a number of the Acts, which have recently passed into law, will make a difference to the rights of children with epilepsy. Among the more significant of these Acts has been the National Disability Authority Act (1999) which is defined as "An act to provide for the establishment of a body to be known as the National Disability Authority." Some of the functions of this Authority are:

a) *"to act as a central, national body which will assist the Minister in the co-ordination and development of policy relating to persons with disabilities;*

b) *to undertake, commission or collaborate in research projects and activities on issues relating to disability and to assist in the development of statistical information appropriate for the planning, delivery and monitoring of programmes and services for persons with disabilities;*

c) *to advise the Minister on appropriate standards for programmes and services provided, or to be provided, to persons with disabilities, and to act as an advisory body with regard to the development of general and specific standards in relation to such programmes and services;*

d) *to monitor the implementation of standards and codes of practice in programmes and services provided to persons with disabilities and to report to the Minister thereon;*

e) *to liaise with other bodies, both corporate and unincorporate, involved in the provision of services to persons with disabilities, and to facilitate and support the development and implementation of appropriate standards for programmes and services for persons with disabilities;"*   [S8.2. (a-e)]

The Act also states that the National Disability Authority shall prepare and submit to the Minister a strategic three year plan, and that the Minister shall, not later than three years after the establishment day, initiate a review of the operation of Parts I and II of the Act. It is hoped that such an Act will provide Brainwave, the Irish Epilepsy Association, with further means of advocacy for people with epilepsy.

Of all the recent Acts it is probably the Education Act (1998) which has the potential for securing the most far reaching benefits for children with epilepsy. However, this Act has serious omissions and ambiguities. The inclusion of the words "where practicable" in many clauses in the Education Act (1998) permits considerable discretion and leeway on the part of the Department of Education and Science. In his review of the Education (No. 2) Bill, the precursor of the 1998 Act, O Murchu (1998) argues that the Bill does not assign the responsibility of delivering a special educational service to any person or authority. Section seven sets down the functions of the Minister in relation to the Act. However, these are broad global functions which deal with planning, co-ordination and provision of support services in a general way, but do not specify the means by which these services will be delivered. Moreover, while the Minister has a duty to provide support services, the manner of the provision creates no entitlement to those services. These services will be provided "as the Minister considers appropriate" [S7.4(b)]. O Murchu (1998) quite rightly states that it is difficult to imagine what this provision does to improve the current, very unsatisfactory situation regarding support services and the lack of entitlement to such services. He also notes that the onus on school authorities to "make reasonable accommodation for students with disabilities" has been weakened in the current Education Act (1998) as the obligation only applies "as the Minister considers appropriate and in accordance with this Act... and within the resources provided to the school." O Murchu (1998) believes that, in including these conditions, the Minister, is in effect, weakening the Constitutional imperative to resource schools effectively. This will have practical implications for children with epilepsy, for example, with regard to such facilities as rooms where they can recover following a seizure. The implementation of the provisions of the Education Act clearly has huge resource and personnel implications, and much of the infrastructure to support certain provisions has yet to be put in place. This will necessitate the training, education, and provision of learning support teachers, career and guidance counsellors, special needs teacher, psychologists, speech therapists, curricular advisors and other support personnel. Effective implementation of the Act will also require considerable in-service training for existing personnel in schools.

Although Glendenning (1999) regards the 1998 Education Act as a singular landmark in Irish education, she believes that while it is neither radical nor prescriptive legislation, its enactment represents a first step in the framing of a wider legislation base for first and second-level education. As such, it formalises, for the first time in the history of the State, a national consensus in education distilled over a nine-year period of intense public debate. In the absence of judicial consideration of the provisions of the Act, Glendenning (1999) takes the view that any analysis of its impact must necessarily be speculative. In the light of cases taken by individuals in the English courts with regard to breach of their Education Acts, Glendenning (1999) is of the opinion that it appears that the Irish courts would be unlikely to hold that the Oireachtas* intended to confer a right on parents to sue for breach of statutory duty under the Education Act 1998. O Murchu (1998) also believes that, even following the precedent established by the O'Donoghue Court Ruling on the educational entitlements of a child with severe mental handicap, and the ensuing review of the Constitution, ambiguities still exist in relation to the right to education for people with special educational needs and how such rights might be safeguarded.

According to Glendenning (1999), the rights of the casualties of the existing system of education to "a certain minimum education" require urgent attention. She believes that little progress can be made unless some definition of "a certain minimum education" is formulated. During submissions to the Constitution Review Group (1996), the Department of Education and Science raised the issue of the definition of "a certain minimum education." It expressed its concern that the absence of a more precise definition of a "certain minimum education" could leave the State vulnerable in enacting any new school attendance legislation that it is seeking to impose a standard which is greater than the minimum as envisaged by the Constitution. Alternatively, it might be argued that the level of education as set by the State is too low. Glendenning (1999) believes that the Department of Education and Science's submission to the Constitution Review Group (1996) indicates a lack of clarity in the definition of a "certain minimum education," and she recommends that the Oireachtas should, as a matter of priority, determine the level of education required as a minimum. However, no such definition has been included in the Education Act (1998), nor in any secondary legislation to date. Glendenning (1999) believes that it is strongly arguable that such an obligation is not merely desirable or concessionary but that it should receive precedence over other, less pressing, educational issues:

> "In the context of limited resources, initiatives to secure the right to "a minimum education" for clearly identified needy groups must gain priority over matters such as free third level fees and ensuring parental preference for alternative school types, where adequate provision already exists" (P.109).

Otherwise, Glendenning (1999) contends that the State may stand accused of discriminating in favour of certain classes of children while denying others their basic constitutional right to a minimum education.

Some European countries such as Finland and Portugal expressly protect the right to special education in their constitutional provisions, whereas other countries have made statutory provision for this. According to Glendenning (1999), international experience generally has shown that separate disability legislation is necessary for effective change in this sphere. Separate legislation has been enacted in the U.S.A. (Americans with Disabilities Act, 1993; Individual with Disabilities Act, 1990), Australia (Disability Discrimination Act, 1992) and Canada (The Act to amend Certain Acts with respect to Persons with Disability 1992, commonly known as the Omnibus Act).

While the O'Donoghue case concerning the rights to a "certain minimum education" vindicated the rights of one child only, Glendenning (1999) believes that it is relevant to all those children who can prove that they have suffered loss or damage at the hands of the State as a consequence of deprivation of their constitutional right to education. As the judge stated:

"…I am satisfied from the evidence in the case that the respondents (the State Department of Education and Science) have failed for some years past to carry out a duty imposed on them by the Constitution to provide for free primary education for his benefit, and for this breach of his constitutional rights that they are liable in damages for any loss and damage thereby caused to the applicant."

It is Glendenning's (1999) belief that this statement has enormous implications for those children who are currently being denied their constitutional right to free primary education, and for other children who can establish that their constitutional rights have been denied or ignored in the past. She considers it necessary to take constitutional action to vindicate this right, but she acknowledges that few parents can afford this investment in time and money. The need for definition of a "certain minimum education" takes on added emphasis for children with epilepsy. Unless this supported minimum entitlement is clearly defined and made accessible by way of supported and resourced pre-school and primary education, the considerable percentage of children with epilepsy who are not availing of any form of education (Brainwave, the Irish Epilepsy Association, 2000) will continue to be denied their Constitutional entitlements.

In the State's appeal against the High Court judgement on the Sinnott Case (2000) concerning what constitutes minimum education for a child with disabilities, the State is now claiming that the High Court judge, Mr. Justice Barr, in directing the State to provide free primary education based on need, not age, has breached the principle of the separation of powers (i.e., between the judiciary and the executive). In the Supreme Court hearing of the State's appeal of the Sinnott Case, Mary Carolan of the Irish Times (2001) reported that Counsel representing the State argued that the High Court's judgement was "..an excessive interference" and that "Mr. Justice Barr was effectively making policy in issuing such an injunction." Counsel for the State further argued that "the High Court was also wrong in the basis on which it awarded damages for breach of Mr. Sinnott's constitutional rights. It would have been sufficient for the judge to declare a breach of constitutional rights in Mr. Sinnott's case – which the State accepted – and to give the State an opportunity to remedy the situation. The judge should have trusted the State to put the matter right." However, it is noteworthy that in recent cases where the High Court has decided that the constitutional requirements of persons with disabilities are not being met, it has in many cases sought to set down what the State must do in order to meet its obligations in respect of provision for free primary education. According to a recent internal report of the Department of Education and Science, under the Chairmanship of the Chief Inspector, Mr. Eamon Stack, entitled A National Support Service for Special Education for Students with Disabilities (2000)*, those who argue for a more interventionist approach by the courts claim this is necessary to ensure that State bodies take appropriate action (e.g. O'Donoghue & O'Hanlon, 2001). However, the Stack Report (2000) also states that, pending any clarification to be made by the Supreme Court, it can be expected that the interventionist approach will be applied in most cases, separation of powers arguments notwithstanding. The Report further states that "..the Department of Education and Science can expect that, for the foreseeable future, the High Court will continue to exert a very considerable influence over individual provision and policy in relation to special education."

Both the recently constituted Governmental Task Forces on Dyslexia and Autism are also indications of a changing climate towards people with special needs in Ireland. It would therefore seem appropriate that Brainwave, the Irish Epilepsy Association, should now press the Department of Education and Science for the establishment of a Task Force on Epilepsy which would examine the educational, social and vocational needs of children with this condition. Undoubtedly however, such initiatives run the risk of securing fragmentary provision for disparate pressure groups. They do not constitute or reflect a coherent policy towards children with special needs, and are not a substitute for a nationally co-ordinated system of special needs education. Up to the present, no Government agency has taken responsibility for ensuring the satisfactory placement of pupils with special needs in Irish schools. Identification, assessment and placement procedures are haphazard, uncoordinated and deteriorating. There is no cohesion between or within Government Departments which share responsibility for the welfare of students with special needs, even where such children attend school. The needs of such pupils are frequently lost sight of in the transition from primary to secondary school. This lack of structure and provision in special needs education is reiterated by Spelman and Kinsella (2000), in the preface to their submission to the Governmental Task Force on Autism, where they state that, "While many worthwhile initiatives in the area of special needs education have been undertaken by Government in recent years, these initiatives have tended to be uncoordinated and fragmentary." This lack of coordinated policy of special needs is further emphasised in the Cromien Report on the internal operation of the State Department of Education and Science, Review of the Department's Operations, Systems and Staffing Needs, as reported in the Irish Independent (Walshe, 2000). The report, undertaken by retired civil servant Sean Cromien at the specific request of the Department of Education and Science, highlighted the shortcomings of an over-centralised Department and recommended urgent reforms.

A Government document, 'Major Initiatives in Special Education Services', which was released by the Minister for Education and Science in October 1998 recognised that all students with disabilities within the mainstream national schools system have an automatic right to support in the form of extra teaching and childcare services. In this document and through various other media outlets, the Minister went to great lengths to point out the "automatic rights" that he had put in place for children with special needs. However, as O'Donoghue and O'Hanlon (2001) quite rightly state, the Minister forgot to mention that this "automatic" right to appropriate education is already enshrined in the Constitution. They also maintain that the Department of Education and Science felt compelled to launch its 'Major Initiatives' Document to counteract the serious and growing liability faced by the State arising from the increasing number of High Court actions asserting its failure to make adequate educational provision for children with special needs. O'Donoghue and O'Hanlon (2001) also contend that the Courts are no longer prepared to tolerate the present inadequate provision for children with special needs and are increasingly directing the State to put the necessary support services in place.

According to the Stack Report (2000), initiatives such as the Government Document, 'Major Initiatives in Special Education Services' (1998), had the effect of temporarily stemming the tide of litigation, but in the past year or so such litigation has resumed with full intensity. This may have prompted the establishment of a Planning Group within the Department of Education and Science under the Chairmanship of Mr. Eamon Stack, Chief Inspector, in October 1999 to review special education provision. The deliberations of the Planning Group were published in November 2000 in the form of a report entitled 'A National Support Service for Special Education for Students with Disabilities'. The Planning Group identified the following challenges which need to be addressed in order for individual students with special educational needs and their parents to gain full access to the necessary services.
- *localised provision of information dissemination, co-ordination and delivery of services*
- *access to appropriate and timely assessment*
- *investigation, research and determination of appropriate response regarding some categories of disability*
- *putting arrangements in place for the delivery of a quality service in an efficient, timely, coherent and non-discriminatory manner and with due regard for local needs*
- *provision of appropriate numbers of adequately trained teachers*
- *provision of a readily accessible, timely and independent appeals mechanism, having due regard to the terms of Section 29 of the Education Act (1998)*

The Stack Report (2000) further recommended that the Minister for Education and Science establish a National Council for Special Education. The Report advocates that the proposed Council should establish a number of Expert Advisory Groups drawn from persons having particular expertise in relation to the category of special need in question, and that a Consultative

Forum should be established in order to facilitate the participation of interest groups in policy formulation.

It is also proposed within the Stack Report (2000), ".. that the Council should exercise a significant information dissemination, co-ordination and delivery role at local level in relation to special needs students." It is recommended that this should be achieved by the Minister for Education and Science initially approving the appointment of 50 Special Needs Organisers (SNO) operating in regional centres. Such SNOs would have the following remit:
- the co-ordination of the provision of special education service in his/her area
- planning in consultation with schools for the inclusion in mainstream education of students with disabilities
- providing a readily available source of information in relation to entitlements of the parents of special needs students in his/her area
- maintaining and ensuring availability of appropriate records, assessment reports etc. in relation to students in his/her area
- ensuring that the progress of students with disabilities is tracked and that it is reviewed at regular specified intervals
- assessing and reviewing the resource requirements in his/her area regarding educational provision for children with disabilities and ensuring that a continuum of special education is available as required in relation to each type of disability

The Stack Report (2000) recognises that the provision of timely and dependable assessment is central to ensuring a comprehensive response to the educational needs of students with disabilities. The establishment of the National Educational Psychological Service (NEPS) and the phased employment of 200 educational psychologists is seen as the key to achieving this objective. It is recommended that, pending the full establishment of NEPS, interim provision should be made to enable schools to source assessment services for the students requiring these. The Report also considers that the final shape of the new structured link between NEPS and the proposed National Council will require consultation with the relevant interest groups and should be considered by the recently established Task Force dealing with the implementation of the Sean Cromien Report 'Review of the Department's Operations, Systems and Staffing Needs'.

The Stack Report (2000) further recommends that the Minister of Education and Science establish an independent forum of appeal in relation to decisions affecting the educational response to the needs of individual special needs children. It is envisaged that the establishment of an Independent Appeal System will reduce the need for recourse to legal proceedings by parents, while also relieving the Special Education Section of the Department of Education and Science of its current involvement in dealing with appeals regarding the adequacy of provision made available for students with disabilities. The Report envisages that, in the future, the Special Education Section will:
- review allocations across the system to ensure an efficient and effective utilisation of resources
- exercise a significant degree of ongoing supervision of the activities of the new support service by putting arrangements in place for regular detailed reports on a national and regional basis from the support service
- identify and agree with the National Council for Special Education on priorities for research into the education of students with disabilities
- collaborate with the Inspectorate in evaluating the overall operation of the system
- concentrate on policy development regarding educational provision for students with disabilities at all levels from pre-school, primary, post-primary, third-level to lifelong learning
- provide advice and information relating to the education of students with disabilities at all levels in the education system. This would include parliamentary questions, adjournment debates, representations and briefings.

One of the most extensive consultation processes ever undertaken by the Irish Government was the National Children's Strategy, the details of which were first published in November 2000. The Strategy sets out an ambitious series of objectives designed to enhance the status and further improve the quality of life of Ireland's children over a ten-year period. It sets three National Goals, one of which guarantees that ".. children will receive quality supports and service to promote all aspects of their development." Of the fourteen objectives associated with this Goal, one refers specifically to children with a disability. It states that they ".. will be entitled to the services they need to achieve their full potential". Under this objective, further proposed actions for persons with a disability include the following:

- A Disabilities Bill which will provide for specific measures to advance and underpin the participation of people with disabilities, in society, including the participation of children with disabilities is being prepared and is expected to be published in 2001.
- Access to services of governmental departments and agencies will be promoted in conjunction with the National Disability Authority. This programme will take all reasonable steps to make public services, including services specific to the needs of children, accessible to people with disabilities within a five year timeframe.
- Key statistical needs in relation to people with disabilities, including children with disabilities, will be reviewed and identified for the purpose of informing policy, planning and delivery of services.
- Supports necessary to enable children with disabilities to obtain a quality education will be developed and participation of students with disabilities in third-level education will be promoted through an access fund.
- Development of a primary pupil database which will allow for more effective identification and response to children with special needs.
- Quality relevant training and placement will be developed to enable young people with disabilities to avail more easily of mainstream employment opportunities and suitable transport and aids and appliances will be provided where their absence is the major barrier to participation in education or training.

Both the National Children's Strategy (2000) and the Stack Report (2000) contain many enlightened and urgently needed recommendations. If properly implemented the proposed initiatives may be the first step in addressing the number of barriers which prevent all pupils with disabilities, including those with epilepsy, gaining full access to quality medical, educational and social services. The proposed establishment of the National Council for Special Education which will provide research and policy advice to the Department of Education and Science is timely and urgently required. However, it is imperative that:

a) the proposed Expert Advisory Groups include persons with particular expertise in relation to the needs of children with epilepsy

b0 the proposed Consultative Forum facilitates the participation of Brainwave, the Irish Epilepsy Association in policy formulation

10.18 SUMMARY

The interview with the Chief Executive of Brainwave, the Irish Epilepsy Association, was conducted to ascertain the applicability and relevance of the study, and in particular the recommendations emanating from the empirical enquiry, to the general wellbeing of children with epilepsy. From the responses, it would appear that all of the recommendations are justifiable and grounded in reality. They are clearly in line with what Brainwave also envisages as being essential if the needs of children with epilepsy are to be addressed by the State.

Although the 1990s have witnessed increased attention to special needs issues in Ireland, Kenny et al. (2000) contend that such developments have been ad hoc and erratic, and there is a general consensus that the provision for pupils with disabilities is very inadequate, both in the development of structures and actual delivery. The situation on the ground, as revealed by the present study, remains little changed in many cases and there is no certainty that children with epilepsy will be included in any of the more recent legislative provisions or policy proposals. It is noticeable, for example, that none of the recent proposals mention epilepsy by name and even the proposals in the Stack Report (2000), refer only to "some categories of disability." There is no doubt that the last decade has witnessed a heightened awareness of the rights of children with special educational needs in Ireland. This is evident in the proliferation of recently enacted legislation seeking to redress the current inadequacies in provision for persons with disabilities and in the increasing number of consultative bodies and discussion documents emanating from or established by central Government. While these initiatives represent enlightened thinking and a heightened awareness of the needs of children with disabilities in Irish society, they are not a substitute for a coherent, co-ordinated national policy for children with special educational needs. Many of the pronouncements of these agencies remain at the aspirational level. There would appear to be much duplication and overlapping in their functions and none of them assumes direct, accountable responsibility for the delivery of services to children with special needs.

The present study has therefore proved to be most successful in providing the first database on children with epilepsy in the Republic of Ireland, and on their parents' experiences of the medical and educational support services in the State. It has revealed some quite fundamental inadequacies in the levels of medical and educational provision and support for children with epilepsy, in comparison with that available in other countries. The recommendations arising from the study are considered to be essential if the rights of children with epilepsy, in common with the rights of children with other special educational needs, are to be upheld as guaranteed by the Constitution and by the Irish Education Act (1998). It is anticipated that the findings of the study will be circulated among key personnel in the Departments of Health and Education and Science. Brainwave, the Irish Epilepsy Association also intends to disseminate the findings and the recommendations among the relevant medical and advisory services. It is hoped in this way that this study, the first of its kind on the problems encountered by children with epilepsy and their parents in Ireland, will help to make the aspirations of the Education Act (1998) and the National Children's Strategy (2000) a tangible reality.

* Both houses of Parliament
* Hereafter referred to as the Stack Report (2000). All quotations from this Report are cited with the express, written permission of the State Department of Education and Science contained in a letter dated 8th June, 2001.

BIBLIOGRAPHY

Aaronson, N. (1988) Quality of life: What is it? How should it be measured? *Oncology*, **2**, 69-74.

Aicardi, J. (1994) *Epilepsy in Children. International Review of Child Neurology Series.* New York: Raven Press.

Aird, R., Masland, R. and Woodbury, D. (1984) *The Epilepsies: A Critical Review*

Aldenkamp, A.P. (1987) Learning difficulties in epilepsy. In: *Education and Epilepsy* (Eds. A.P. Aldenkamp, W.C.J. Alpheerts, H. Meinardi and G. Stores) Swaets and Zeitlinger Lisse (NL) Berwyn USA.

Aldenkamp *et al.* (1989), Learning Disabilities in Epliepsy. In: Aldenkamp A.P. and Alpheerts W.C.J., Meinardi H. and Stores G., (Eds), *Education and Epilepsy,* Swets and Zeitlinger Lesse, (NL) Berwyn USA.

Aldenkamp, A.P., Alpherts, W.C.J., Blennow, G., *et al.* (1993) Withdrawal of antiepileptic medication in children – effects on cognitive function: The Multicenter Holmfrid Study. *Neurology* **43**:41-50.

America (1990) Individual's with Disabilities Act. US Government Printing Office

America (1993) Americans with Disabilities Act. US Government Printing Office

Andermann, L. and Andermann, F. (1992) University students with epilepsy: a study of social aspects. *Seizure* **1**: 173-176.

Anderson, E. and Barton, R. (1990) Epilepsy- a family burden? *Clinical Psychology Forum* **25**, 3-6.

Andrews, D.G., Bullen, J.G., Tomlinson, L. *et al.* (1986) A comparative study of the cognitive effects of phenytoin and carbamazepine in new referrals with epilepsy. *Epilepsia* **27**: 128-134.

Appolone, C. (1978) Preventative social work intervention with families of children with epilepsy. *Social Work and Health Care* **4**: 139-148.

Arangio, A. (1980) The social worker and epilepsy: A description of assessment and treatment variables. In: *A Multidisciplinary Handbook of Epilepsy* (Ed. B.P. Hermann). Springfield IL, Charles C. Thomas.

Austin, J.K., Shelton Smith M., Risinger, M.W., McNelis, A.M. (1994) Childhood epilepsy and asthma: comparison of quality of life. *Epilepsia* **35**: 608-615.

Australia (1992) Disability Discrimination Act. Australia Government Printing Office.

Bagley, C. (1971) *The Social Psychology of the Child with Epilepsy* London, Routledge and Kegan Paul.

Bagley, C. (1972) Social prejudice and the adjustment of people with epilepsy. *Epilepsia* **13**: 33-45.

Baker, G.A., Jacoby, A., Buck, D., Stalgis, C. and Monnet, D. (1997) Quality of life of people with epilepsy:a European study. *Epilepsia* **38**(3): 353-362.

Bannon, M.J., Wildig, C. and Jones, P.W. (1992) Teachers' perceptions of epilepsy. *Archives of Disease in Childhood*, **67**: 1467-1471.

Baumann, R.J., Wilson, J.E. and Wiese, H.J. (1995) Kentuckians' attitudes towards children with epilepsy. *Epilepsia* **36**: 1003-8.

Beech, L. (1992) Knowledge of epilepsy among relatives of the epilepsy sufferer. *Seizure* **1**: 133-135.

Bell, J. (1993) *Doing Your Research Project, A Guide for First-Time Researchers in Education and Social Science,* 2nd Edition, Bucks. O.U.P.

Berkovic, S.F., Howell, R.A., Hay, D.A. and Hopper, J.L. (1998) Epilepsies in twins: genetics of the major epilepsy syndromes. *Annals of Neurology.* Vol.43 No. 4. P. 435-445.

Berrios, G.E. (1984) Epilepsy and insanity during the early 19th century. *Archives in Neurology,* **41,** 978-981.

Besag, F.M.C. (1987) The role of a special school for children with epilepsy. In: *Epilepsy and Education* (Eds. J. Oxley and G. Stores). The Medical Tribune Group.

Besag, F.M.C. (1988a) *Schooling the Child with Epilepsy. The Royal College of General Practitioners Members' Reference Book, 370-372,* London RCGP.

Besag, F.M.C. (1988b) Which school for the child with epilepsy? *Med, 2*; (2), 16-17.

Besag, F.M.C., Loney, G., Waudby, E. *et al.* (1989b) A multidisciplinary approach to epilepsy, learning difficulties and behavioural problems. *Journal of Educational and Child Psychology* **6** (2): 18-24.

Besag, F.M.C. (1993) Epilepsy, learning and behaviour: an overview. *Journal of Educational and Child Psychology* **10** (1): 36-45.

Besag, F.M.C. (1994) Epilepsy, education and the role of mental handicap. In *Epilepsy and Education* Vol. 2, No. 3: 561-583 (Eds. E.M. Ross and R.C. Woody) Balliere's Clinical Paediatrics International Practice and Research.

Besag, F.M.C. (1995) Epilepsy, Learning and Behaviour in Childhood. *Epilepsia,* **36** (Suppl. 1):S58-S63.

Betts, T. (1993) Neuropsychiatry. In: Laidlaw J., Richens, A. and Chadwick, D. (Eds.) *A Textbook of Epilepsy* Edinburgh, Churchill, Livingstone.

Boreham, P. and Gibson, D. (1978) The informative process in private medical consultations: A preliminary investigation. *Social Science and Medicine* **15b:** 409-416.

Bourgeois, B.F.D., Prensky, A.L., Palkes, H.S., Talent, B.K and Busch, S.G., (1983) Intelligence in epilepsy: a prospective study in children *Annals of Neurology,* **14,** 438-444.

Brainwave, The Irish Epilepsy Association (1998) *Your Guide to Epilepsy* (Information Booklet).

Brainwave, The Irish Epilepsy Association (1991) Submission to the Review Committee on Special Education (Unpublished).

Brainwave, The Irish Epilepsy Association (1991) A Teacher's Guide (Information Booklet).

Brainwave, The Irish Epilepsy Association (1992) *Explaining Epilepsy.* (Information Booklet).

Brainwave, The Irish Epilepsy Association. (1992) *Seizures* (Information Booklet).

Brainwave, The Irish Epilepsy Association (1992) *Epilepsy. Questions and Answers.* (Information Booklet).

Brainwave, The Irish Epilepsy Association (1992) *A Teacher's Guide* (Information Booklet).

Brainwave, The Irish Epilepsy Association (1998) Special Exam Considerations for State Examinations In: *Epilepsy News.* The Irish Epilepsy Association.

Brainwave, The Irish Epilepsy Association (2000) Doctors' Pack. The Irish Epilepsy Association.

Brent, D.A., Crumrine, P.K., Varma, R. *et al.* (1990) Phenobarbital treatment and major depressive disorder in children with epilepsy: a naturalistic follow-up. *Pediatrics,* **85,** 1086-1091.

Brett, E.M. and Neville, B.G.R. (1997) Epilepsy and convulsions: the surgical treatment of epilepsy in childhood. In: *Paediatric Neurology*. (Ed. Brett E.M.) Edinburgh: Churchill Livingstone.

British Epilepsy Association (1995) *Epilepsy and Education* (Information Booklet).

Brodie, M.J., Shorvon, D., Johannessen, S., Halasz, P., Reynolds, E.H., Wieser, H.G. and Wolf, P. (1997) Appropriate standards of epilepsy care across Europe. *Epilepsia*, 38, 1245-50.

Browne, T.R. (1983) Antiepileptic drugs and psychosocial development: ethosuximide. In: *Antiepileptic Drug Therapy in Pediatrics* (Eds. P.L. Morselli, C.E. Pippenger and J.K. Penry), Raven Press, New York, pp. 181-187.

Came, F., and Webster V. (1988*) Special Educational Needs in Mainstream Schools: A Head's Guide*, ISC, Learning Works.

Camfield, P.R., Gates, R., Ronen, G. *et al.* (1984) Comparison of cognitive ability, personality profile and school success in epileptic children with pure right versus left temporal lobe EEG foci. *Annals of Neurology*, 15, 122-126.

Canada (1992) The Act to Amend Certain Acts with Respect to Persons with Disability (Omnibus Act).

Canger, R. and Cornaggia, C. (1985) Public attitudes towards epilepsy in Italy: results of a survey and comparison with U.S.A. and West German data. *Epilepsia* 26: 221-6.

Carolan, M. (March, 2001) *State Tells Court Free Education Only for Children*. Irish Times.

Carpay, H.A., Vermeulen, J., Stroink, H., Brouwer, O.F., Boudewyn Peters, A.C., van Donselaar, C.A., Aldenkamp, A.P. and Arts, W.F.M. (1997) Disability due to restrictions in childhood epilepsy. *Developmental Medicine and Child Neurology* 39: 521-526.

Carroll, D. (1992) Employment among young people with epilepsy. *Seizure* 1: 127-131.

Caveness, W.E. and Gallup, G.S. (1980) A survey of public attitudes towards epilepsy in 1979 with an indication of trends over the past thirty years. *Epilepsia* 21: 509-18.

Chadwick, D. (1990) Diagnosis of epilepsy. *Lancet*, 336, 291-5.

Chaplin, J.E., Yepez Lasso, R., Shorvon, S.D. and Floyd, M. (1992) National general practice study of epilepsy: the social and psychological effects of a recent diagnosis of epilepsy. *British Medical Journal* 304:1416-18.

Chappell, B. (1992) Epilepsy: patient views on their condition and treatment. *Seizure* 1, 103-109.

Chen, Y.J., Kang, W.M., Chin-Mino, So.W. (1996) Comparison of antiepileptic drugs on cognitive function in newly diagnosed epileptic children: a psychometric and neurophysiological study. *Epilepsia* 37: 81-6.

Chung, M.Y., Chang, Y.C., Lai, Y.H.C. and Lai, C.W. (1995) Survey of public awareness, understanding, and attitudes toward epilepsy in Taiwan. *Epilepsia*, 36 (5): 488-493.

Clancy, M. (1998) My Story. In: *Epilepsy News*, Brainwave, the Irish Epilepsy Association.

Clare, M., Aldridge Smith, J. and Wallace, S.J. (1978) A. child's first febrile convulsion. *Practitioner*, 221: 775-776.

Colgan, P. (March, 2000) Epilepsy waiting times in Ireland set to double. *The Sunday Times.*

Commission for the Control of Epilepsy and its Consequences (1978) *Plan for Nationwide Action on Epilepsy*, Vol. II DHEW Publication no. 78-279. Bethesda, MD.

Commission on Classification and Terminology of the International League Against Epilepsy (1981) Proposal for revised clinical and electroencephalographic classification of epileptic seizures. *Epilepsia,* **22**, 489-501.

Commission on Classification and Terminology of the International League Against Epilepsy (1985) Proposal for classification of epilepsy and epileptic syndromes. *Epilepsia,* **26**, 268-278.

Commission on Classification and Terminology of the International League against Epilepsy (1989) Proposal for revised classification of epilepsies and epileptic syndromes. *Epilepsia,* **30**, 389-399.

Constitution of Ireland (1937) Dublin: Government Publications.

Coolahan J. (1981) *Irish Education: Its History and Structure.* Dublin Institute of Public Administration.

Cox, B. *et al.* (1987) The Health and Lifestyle Survey: Preliminary Report of a Nationwide Survey of the Physical and Mental Health Attitudes: Attitudes and Lifestyles of a Random Sample of 9003 British Adults: Health Promotion Trust.

Craig, A. and Oxley, J. (1988) Social aspects of epilepsy. In: *A Textbook of Epilepsy* (Eds. J. Laidlaw, A.Richens, J.Oxley) Edinburgh, Churchill Livingstone.

Cromien, S. (2000) *Review of the Department's Operations, Systems and Staffing Needs.* (Unpublished Department of Education and Science Internal Document).

Cull, C.A. and Brown, S.W. (1989) The education of children with epilepsy in the U.K. In: *Epilepsy and Education: Policies for the Child with Epilepsy* (Eds. A.P. Aldenkamp, A. Das Gupta and V.S. Saxena) The International Bureau for Epilepsy.

Daly, T. (2000) Context and assistive technology in Irish mainstream education. A paper presented at a conference on *Human Factors in Delivering an Assistive Technology Service: from Local to Global.* Central Remedial Clinic, Dublin. (Publication pending)

Dam, M. and Gram, L. (1986) *Epilepsy – Prejudice and Fact.* London, Chapman and Hall.

de Boer, H.M., Aldenkamp, A.P., Bullivant, F. *et al.* (1994) Horizon: the transnational epilepsy training project. *Int. J. Adolescent Med. Heal.* 7:325-35.

de Boer, H.M. (1995) Epilepsy and society. *Epilepsia* 36 (Suppl.1):S8-S11.

de Jong, P., Stravens, W., Kuip, J. and Harms, T. (1997) Children with Epilepsy: Regular or Special Education "de Berkenschutse"/de Waterlelie" Special Schools for Children with Epilepsy. Poster Presentation, International Congress.

Department of Education, England (1941) Education after the War – A Green Paper. HMSO.

Department of Education and Science, England (1978) Special Educational Needs. Report of the Committee of Enquiry into the Education of Handicapped Children and Young People. Chair: Warnock H.M., HMSO: London.

Department of Education, Ireland (1994) Directory of Special Schools, Dublin, S.O.

Department of Education, Ireland (1996) Charting our Educational Future: White Paper on Education. Dublin: S.O.

Department of Education and Science, Ireland (1998) A National Educational Psychological Service. Report of Planning Group. Dublin S.O.

Department of Education and Science, Ireland (1998) Major Initiatives in Special Education Services. Dublin S.O.

Department of Education and Science, Ireland (1999) Special Educational Needs: Curriculum Issues, Discussion Paper. National Council for Curriculum and Assessment. Dublin: S.O.

Department of Education and Science, Ireland (1999) Task Force on Dyslexia

Department of Education and Science, Ireland (1999) Task force on Autism

Department of Education and Science, Ireland (2000) *The Report of the Expert Advisory Group on Certificate Examinations (2000)*. Arrangements for the Assessment of Candidates with Special Needs in Certificate Examinations. Report to the Minister for Education and Science. Dublin S.O.

Department of Education and Science, Ireland (November, 2000) A National Support Service for Special Education for Students with Disabilities. Report of a Planning Group under the Chairmanship of Mr. Eamon Stack, Chief Inspector. (Unpublished Internal Document).

Department of Health, Ireland (1936) Commission of Enquiry into the Reformation and Industrial School System, Dublin S.O.

Department of Health, Ireland (1965) Commission of Enquiry on Mental Handicap, Dublin S.O.

Department of Health and Social Security and Welsh Office (1969) People with Epilepsy (Report of a joint sub-committee of the Standing Medical Advisory Committee on the health and welfare of handicapped persons). Her Majesty's Stationery Office, London.

Dell, J.L. (1986) Social dimensions of epilepsy: stigma and response. In: *Psychopathology in Epilepsy*. (Eds. S. Whitman, B.P. Herman) New York: Oxford University Press, p.185-210.

Dinnage, R. (1986) *The Child with Epilepsy*. National Children's Bureau Bibliographies

Dodrill, C.B. (1986) Correlates of generalized tonic-clonic seizures with neuropsychological, emotional and social functioning in parents with epilepsy . *Epilepsia*. 27:399-411.

Dodrill, C. B., and Temkin, N.R. (1989) Motor speed is a contaminating factor in evaluating the cognitive effects of phenytoin. *Epilepsia* **30**: 453-7.

Duncan, J. (1990) Medical factors affecting the quality of life in patients with epilepsy. In: Chadwick, D. (Ed.) *The Quality of Life and the Quality of Care in Epilepsy*. London: Royal Society of Medicine.

Education, Science and Arts Committee (1987) *Special Education Needs: Implementation of the Education Act 1981*, Volume **1**. Third Report, session 1986-87, HMSO London.

Egg-Olofsson, O. (1985) Types of epilepsy in the young schoolchild: stress, flicker and nocturnal seizures. In: *Paediatric Perspectives on Epilepsy* (Eds. E. Ross and E. Reynolds) John Wiley and Sons Ltd.

Egg-Olofsson, O. (1990) Basic principles of the classifications of epileptic seizures and syndromes. In *Paediatric Epilepsy* (Eds. M. Sillanpaa, S.I. Johannessen, G. Blennow and M.Dam) Wrightson Biomedical Publishing Ltd.

Ellenberg, J.H., Hirtz, D.G. and Nelson, K.B. (1985) Do seizures in children cause intellectual deterioration? *Annals of Neurology* **18**: 389.

Engel, J. (1989) *Seizures and Epilepsy*. Philadelphia: FA Davis.

Engel, J. (1995) Concepts of epilepsy. *Epilepsia*, **36**, (Suppl. 1):S23-S29.

European Social Fund Evaluation (1996) Evaluation Report: Early Leavers.

Ferrari, M., Matthews, W.S. and Barabas, G. (1983) The family and the child with epilepsy. *Family Process* **22**: 53-59.

Finke, M. (1980) Public attitudes towards epilepsy in the Federal Republic of Germany: trends over the past decade. *Epilepsia* **21**: 201-2.

Floyd, M. (1986) A review of published studies on epilepsy and employment. In: *Epilepsy and Employment* (Ed. J. Oxley). London, Royal Society of Medicine.

Floyd, M., Chaplin, J. and Lisle, J. (1993) Pre-employment screening of NHS employees with epilepsy. *Occupational Medicine* **43**, 193-6.

Freeman, J.M. (1987) A clinical approach to the child with seizures and epilepsy. *Epilepsia,* **28**, (Suppl.) 103-9.

Gale, J.L., Thapa, P.B., Wassilak, S.G.F. *et al.* (1994) Risk of serious acute neurological illness after immunisation with Diphtheria-Pertussis-Tetanus vacinne. *Journal of the American Medical Association* **271**, 37-41.

Gastaut, H. (1965) Enquiry into the education of epileptic children. In: *Epilepsy and Education: Report on a seminar in Marseilles,* April 1964, British Epilepsy Association and International Bureau for Epilepsy, p.3.

Gastaut, H. (1970) Clinical and electroencephalographical classifications of epileptic seizures. *Epilepsia* **11**, 102-113.

Gastaut, H. (1973) *Dictionary of Epilepsy,* World Health Organisation, Geneva.

Geurrant, J., Anderson, W.W. and Fischer, A. *et al.* (1962) *Personality in Epilepsy* Thomas Springfield.

Giordani, B., Berent, S., Sackellares, J.C. *et al.* (1985) Intelligence test performance of patients with partial and generalized seizures. *Epilepsia,* **26**: 37-42.

Glendenning, D. (1999) *Education and the Law.* Butterworths (Ireland) Ltd.

Glowinski, H. (1973) Cognitive deficits in temporal lobe epilepsy. *Journal of Nervous and Mental Disorders* **157**: 129-137.

Good News Bible, Today's English Version (1976) *Mark* Chapter 9 (v: 17-29).

Goodridge, D.M.G. and Shorvon, S.D. (1983) Epileptic seizures in a population of 6000. 1. Demography, diagnosis and role of the hospital services. 2. Treatment and prognosis. *British Medical Journal* **287**, 641-7.

Gordon, N. and Sillanpaa, M. (1997) Epilepsy and prejudice with particular relevance to childhood. *Developmental Medicine and Child Neurology* **39**: 777-781.

Grant, R. (1981) Special Centres. In: *Epilepsy and Psychiatry* (Eds. E.R. Reynolds and M.R. Trimble) Edinburgh: Churchill-Livingstone.

Great Britain, (1899) Elementary Education (Defective and Epileptic Children) Act HMSO, London.

Great Britain, (1918) Education Act HMSO, London.

Great Britain, (1921) Education Act HMSO, London.

Great Britain, (1944) Education Act HMSO, London.

Great Britain (1970) Handicapped Act HMSO, London

Great Britain, (1945) Health and Handicapped Pupils' Regulations HMSO, London.

Great Britain, (1981) Education Act, HMSO, London.

Great Britain, (1993) Education Act, London DES.

Green, S. (1985) Counselling the parent of the child with epilepsy. In: *Paediatric Perspectives on Epilepsy* (Eds. E. Ross and E. Reynolds) John Wiley & Sons Ltd.

Green, J.B. and Hartlage, L. (1970) 'Comparative performance of epileptic and non-epileptic children and adolescents on academic, communicative and social skills' (Abstract) 3rd European Symposium on Epilepsy. Marienlyst.

Green, J.B. and Hartlage, L.C. (1971) Comparative performance of epileptic and non-epileptic children and adolescents. *Diseases of the Nervous System* **32**:418-421.

Gudmundsson, G. (1966) Epilepsy in Iceland. *Acta Neurol. Scand.*, **43** (suppl.), 25.

Guey, J., Charles, C., Coquery, C., Roger, J., Soulayrol, R. (1967) Study of psychological effects of ethosuximide (Zarontin) on 25 children suffering from petit mal epilepsy. *Epilepsia*, **8**, 129.

Gunn, J. (1981) Medico-Legal Aspects of Epilepsy. In: *Epilepsy and Psychiatry* (Eds. E.H. Reynolds and M.R. Trimble) Churchill Livingstone, Edinburgh.

Hall, B., Martin, E. and Smithson, H. (1997) *Epilepsy, A General Practice Problem.* The Royal College of General Practitioners.

Hanai, T. (1996) Quality of life in children with epilepsy. *Epilepsia*, **37** (Suppl. 3):28-32.

Hartlage, L.C. and Green, J.B. (1972) The relation of parental attitudes to academic and social achievement in epileptic children. *Epilepsia*, **13**, 21-26.

Hauser, W.A. (1994) The distribution of mild and severe forms of epilepsy. In: *Epilepsy and Quality of Life* (Eds. M.R. Trimble and W.E. Dodson) New York: Raven Press.

Hauser, W.A. (1978) Epidemiology of epilepsy. In: *Advances in Neurology*, (Ed. Schoenberg, B.C.) vol. **19**, 313-339. Raven Press, New York.

Hauser, W.A. and Anderson, V.E. (1986) Genetics of epilepsy. In: *Recent Advances in Epilepsy*, No. 3 (Eds. T.A. Pedley and B.S. Meldrum), Churchill Livingstone, Edinburgh, London.

Hauser, W.A., Annegers, J.F. and Anderson, V.E. (1983) Epidemiology and the genetics of epilepsy. In: *Epilepsy* (Eds. A. A. Ward, J. R. Penry and D. Purpura) Raven Press, New York.

Helgeson, D.C., Mittan, R., Tan, S. and Chayasirisobhon, S. (1990) Sepulveda epilepsy education: The efficacy of a psychoeducational treatment programme in treating medical and psychosocial aspects of epilepsy. *Epilepsia* **31**: 75-82.

Henriksen, G.F. (1972) The role of special centres in the care of epileptics in Norway. *Epilepsia* **13**: 199-204.

Herranz, J.L., Arteaga, R. and Armijo, J.A. (1982) Side effects of sodium valporate in monotherapy controlled by plasma levels: a study of 88 paediatric patients. *Epilepsia*, **23**, 203-14.

Hicks, R.A., and Hicks, M.J., (1991) Attitudes of major employers toward the employment of people with epilepsy: a 30 year study. *Epilepsia*: **32** (1): 86-88.

Hill, D. (1981) Historical Review. In: *Epilepsy and Psychiatry* (Eds. E.H. Reynolds and M.R. Trimble) Churchill Livingstone, Edinburgh.

Hoare, P. (1984a) Psychiatric disturbance in the families of epileptic children. *Developmental Medicine and Child Neurology* **26**: 14-19.

Hoare, P. (1984b) Does illness foster dependency? A study of epileptic and diabetic children. *Developmental Medicine and Child Neurology* **26**: 14-19

Hoare. P. (1986) Adults' attitudes to children with epilepsy: The use of a visual analogue scale questionnaire. *Journal of Psychosomatic Research* **30**: 471-479.

Hoare, P. (1993) The quality of life of children with chronic epilepsy and their families. *Seizure, 2*, 269-275.

Hoare, P. and Russell, M. (1995) The quality of life of children with chronic epilepsy and their families: Preliminary findings with a new assessment measure. *Developmental Medicine and Child Neurology* **37**, 689-696.

Hoare, P. and Kerley, S. (1991) Psychosocial adjustment of children with chronic epilepsy and their families. *Developmental Medicine and Child Neurology* **33**: 201-215.

Holdsworth, L. and Whitmore, K. (1971) Some observations from a study of children with epilepsy who were attending ordinary schools. *Spastics Study Group on Medical Aspects of Children with School Difficulties, Durham.*

Holdsworth, L. and Whitmore, K. (1974) A study of children with epilepsy attending ordinary schools. I: Their seizure patterns, progress and behaviour in schools. *Developmental Medicine and Child Neurology,* **36**, 746-758.

Holdsworth, L. and Whitmore, K. (1974b) A study of children with epilepsy attending ordinary schools. II: Information and attitudes held by their teachers. *Developmental Medicine and Child Neurology,* **16**, 759-765.

Hopkins, A. (1983) *Epilepsy in Adults.* Medicine International.

Hopkins, A. (1987) Prescribing in pregnancy – Epilepsy and anticonvulsant drugs. *British Medical Journal* **294**:497-500.

Hopkins, A. (1995) The causes of epilepsy, the risk factors for epilepsy and the precipitation of seizures. In: *Epilepsy* (Eds. Hopkins, A., Shorvon, S. and Cascino, G.) London, Chapman and Hall.

Houston, M. (November, 2000) Hospital Waiting Times. The Irish Times

Hutt, S.J., Jackson, R.M., Belsham, A. and Higgins, G. (1968) Perceptual-motor behaviour in relation to blood phenobarbitone level: A preliminary report. *Developmental Medicine and Child Neurology,* **10**, 626-632

Iivanainen, M., Uutela, A. and Vilkkumaa, I. (1980) Public awareness and attitudes towards epilepsy in Finland. *Epilepsia,* **21**:413-23.

Iliff, A. (1998) Liar: film review. *International Epilepsy News* No.132.

Ingwell R.H. Toreson, R.W., and Smith, S.J. (1967) Accuracy of social perception if physically handicapped and non-handicapped persons. *Journal of Social Psychology.* **22**:107-116.

Ireland (1980) A White Paper on Educational Development. Dublin S.O.

Ireland (1983) The Education and Training of Severely Mentally Handicapped Children in Ireland. Report of a Working Party to the Minister for Education and the Minister for Health and Social Welfare. Dublin S.O.

Ireland (1990) Report of the Primary Education Review Body, Dublin S.O.

Ireland (1991) Child Care Act. Dublin S.O.

Ireland (1993) Report of the Special Education Review Committee: Dublin, S.O.

Ireland (1996) A Strategy for Equality: Report of the Commission on the Status of People with Disabilities. Dublin: Department of Equality and Law Reform.

Ireland (1996) Constitution Review Group. Dublin S.O.

Ireland (1997a) Education Bill. Dublin S.O.

Ireland (1997b) Education (No.2) Bill. Dublin S.O.

Ireland (1998) Education Act. Dublin S.O.

Ireland (1999) Education (Welfare) Bill. Dublin S.O.

Ireland (1999) National Disability Authority Act. Dublin: S.O.

Ireland (1999) White Paper on Early Childhood Education. Dublin S.O.

Ireland (2000) Education (Welfare) Act. Dublin S.O.

Ireland (2000) Equal Status Act. Dublin S.O.

Ireland (2000) The National Children's Strategy. Dublin: S.O.

Jacoby, A. and Chadwick, D. (1992) Psychosocial problems in epilepsy. *British Medical Journal* **305**:117 (Letter).

Jarvie, S., Espie, C.A. and Brodie, M.J. (1993) The development of a questionnaire to assess knowledge of epilepsy: 1-general knowledge of epilepsy. *Seizure* **2**: 179-185.

Jarvie, S., Espie, C.A. and Brodie, M.J. (1993) The development of a questionnaire to assess knowledge of epilepsy: 2- knowledge of own condition. *Seizure* **2**: 187-193.

Jenson, R. and Dam, M. (1992) Public attitudes towards epilepsy in Denmark. *Epilepsia* **33**: 459-63.

Joensen, P. (1986) Prevalence, incidence and classification of epilepsy in the Faroes. *Acta Neurol. Scand.* **74**, 150-155

Kangesu, E., McGowan, M.E.L. and Edeh, J. (1984) Management of epilepsy in schools. *Archives of Diseases in Childhood*, **59**, 45-47.

Kenny, M. *et al.* (2000) *Hidden Voices* Bradshaw Books, Cork

Kerry Network of People with Disabilities in Ireland (2000) *Visualising Inclusion*

Krohn, W. (1961) A study of epilepsy in Northern Norway, its frequency and characteristics. *Acta Psychol. Neurol. Scand.* (suppl.), **150**, 215-225.

Kugoh, T. and Hosokawa, K. (1991) Psychological aspects of patients with epilepsy and their family members. *Epilepsia*: **32** (suppl. 1):43.

Kurtz, G. (1983) Special schooling for children with epilepsy In: *Research Progress in Epilepsy* (Ed. F.C. Rose) Pitman: London.

Lai, C.W., Huang, X., Lai, Y.H.C., Zhang, Z., Liu, G. and Yang, M.Z. (1990) Survey of public awareness, understanding, and attitudes toward epilepsy in Henan Province China. *Epilepsia* **31**: 182-7.

LaMartina, J.M. (1989) Uncovering public misconceptions about epilepsy. *Journal of Epilepsy* **2**: 45-8.

Leviton, A. and Cowan, L.D. (1982) Methodoligical issues in the epidemiology of seizure disorders in children. *Neuropidemiology*, **1**,40-83.

Lund, M. and Randrup, J. (1972) A day-centre for severely handicapped people with epilepsy. *Epilepsia* **13**: 245-247.

Lebrun, Y. (1992) The language of epilepsy. *Seizure* **1**:207-212.

Lennox, W.G. and Lennox, M.A. (1960) *Epilepsy and Related Disorders.* Little Brown, Boston.

Leviton, A. and Cowan, L.D. (1982) Epidemiology of seizure disorders in children. *Neuroepidemiology,* **1**, 40-83.

Long, C.G. and Moore, J.R. (1979) Parental expectations for their epileptic children. *Journal of Child Psychology and Psychiatry* **20**, 4, 299-312.

Lothman, D.J. (1990) Mother child interactions in children with epilepsy: relations with child competence. *Journal of Epilepsy* **3**: 157-163.

MacFarlane, A. (1992) 'Personal child health records' held by parents. *Archives of Disease in Childhood* **67**: 571-2.

McDonnell, P., (1992) Vested Interests in the Development of Special Education in Ireland, *Reach*, Vol **5**, 2, 97-106.

McGee, P., (1990) Special Education in Ireland. *European Journal of Special Needs in Education.* 5.1.,48-64.

McLellan, D.L. (1987) Epilepsy and employment. *Journal of the Society of Occupational Medicine* **37**: 94-99.

McKusick, V.A. (1983) Mendelian inheritance in man. *Catalogs of Autosomal Dominant, Autosomal Recessive and X-Linked Phenotypes,* 6th Edition, John Hopkins University Press, Baltimore.

McLin, W.M. and de Boer, H.M. (1995) Public perceptions about epilepsy. *Epilepsia* **36**(10): 957-959.

Mc Menamin, J. and O'Connor Bird, M. (1997) *Epilepsy, A Parent's Guide.* Brainwave, The Irish Epilepsy Association.

Maj, M., Del Veechio, M., Tata, M.R., Guizzaro, A., Bravaccio, F. and Kamali, D. (1987) Perceived parental rearing behaviour and psychopathology in epileptic patients: A controlled study. *Psychopathology* **20**: 196-202.

Matthews, J. (1983) The communication process in clinical settings. *Social Science and Medicine* **17**: 1371-1378.

Meador, K.J., Loring, D.W., Huh, K. *et al.* (1990) Comparative cognitive effects of anticonvulsants. *Neurology,* **40**: 391-4.

Meinardi, H. (1972) Special centres in The Netherlands. *Epilepsia* **13**:191-197.

Mellor, D.H. and Lowitt, I. (1977) In: *Epilepsy: The Eight International Symposium.* (Ed. Penry, J.K.) New York: Raven Press.

Morgan, J. and Kurtz, Z. (1987) *Special Services for People with Epilepsy* HMSO: London.

Morrow, J.I. (1993) Specialised epilepsy clinic — the pros and cons. *Seizure* **2**: 267-268.

Mitchell, W.G., Schneider, L.M. and Baker, S.A. (1994) Psychosocial behavioural and medical outcomes in children with epilepsy: a developmental risk factor model using longitudinal data. *Pediatrics* **94**: 471-7.

Mittan, R.J. (1986) Fear of seizures. In: *Epilepsy: Social Dimensions* (Eds. B. Hermann and S. Whitman) Oxford, Oxford University Press.

Needham, W.E. *et al.* (1969) Intelligence and EEG studies in families with idiopathic epilepsy. *Journal of the American Medical Association,* **207**, 8, 1497-1501.

Nelson, K.B. and Ellenberg, J.H. (1987) Predisposing and causative factors in childhood epilepsy. *Epilepsia,* **28,** Suppl. 1. S.16-S.24.

O'Connor, R., Cox, J. and Coughlan, M. (1992) *Guidelines for the Diagnosis and Management of Epilepsy in General Practice.* Irish College of General Practitioners.

O'Donohue, N.V. (1983) What should the child with epilepsy be allowed to do? *Archives of Disease in Childhood* **58**:934-7.

O'Donohue, N.V. (1985) *Epilepsies of Childhood* Butterworth-Heinemann Ltd.

O'Donohue, N.V. (1994) *Epilepsies of Childhood* Butterworth-Heinemann Ltd.

O'Donoghue, M. and O'Hanlon, P. (2001) *A Guide to Your Child's Educational Entitlements.* Information Campaign: The Association for the Severely and Profoundly Mentally Handicapped.

Office of the Ombudsman (1998) Enquiry into the Department of Education School Transport System.

Oliver, E. (November, 2000) Measures to assist autistic children planned. *The Irish Times.*

O' Murchu, E. (1998) Education (No.2) bill: where are the guarantees? *Reach Journal of Special Needs in Ireland,* Vol. 11 No.**2**, 76-81.

O' Toole, J. (1998) Are our children special? In: *In Touch,* Irish National Teachers' Organisation.

Ounsted, C., Lindsay, J., Norman, R. (1966) Biological factors in temporal lobe epilepsy. *Clinics in Developmental Medicine* No.**22** London: S.I.M.P. with Heinemann Medical.

Pachlatko, C. (1993) Economic aspects of epilepsy. *Epilepsia* **34**: (Suppl. 2) :137.

Paladin, A.V. (1995) Epilepsy in twentieth century literature. *Epilepsia* **36**: 1058-60.

Pazzaglia, P. and Frank-Pazzaglia, L. (1976) Record in grade school of pupils with epilepsy: an epidemiological study. *Epilepsia* **17**: 361-366

Pond, H. (1979) Parental attitudes towards children with a chronic medical disorder: special reference to diabetes mellitus. *Diabetes Care* **2**:425-431.

Pond, D. (1981) Psycho-social aspects of epilepsy - the family. In: *Epilepsy and Psychiatry* (Trimble, M.R. and Reynolds, E.H.) Churchill Livingstone.

Rantakallio, P. and von Wendt, L. (1986) A prospective comparative study of the aetiology of cerebral palsy and epilepsy in a one-year birth cohort from Northern Finland. *Acta Paediatr. Scand.* **75**, 586-592.

Reiner, W.O., (1982) Restreictive Factors in the education of children with epilepsy from a medical point of view. In: Aldenkamp, A.P., Alphert, W.E.J., Meincudi, H., Stores, G.

Remy, C. and Beaumont, D. (1989) Efficacy and safety of vigabatrin in the long-term treatment of refractory epilepsy. *British Journal of Clinical Pharmacology,* **27**, Supplement 1, S125-S129.

Reynolds, E.H. (1989) Historical Aspects. In: *Epilepsy, Behaviour and Cognitive Function* (Eds. M.R. Trimble and E.H. Reynolds).

Ritchie, K. (1981) Interaction in families of epileptic children. *Journal of Child Psychology and Psychiatry* **22**: 65-71.

Rocca, W.A., Sharbrough, F.W., Hauser, W.A., Annegers, J.F. and Schoeberg, B.S. (1987a) Risk factors for complex partial seizures: A population-based case-control study. *Annals of Neurology* **21**, 22-31.

Rocca, W.A., Sharbrough, F.W., Hauser, W.A., Annegers, J.F. and Schoeberg, B.S. (1987c) Risk factors for absence seizures: A population-based case-control study in Rochester, Minnesota. *Neurology,* **37**, 1309-1314.

Rogan, P. (1980) *Epilepsy A Teacher's Handbook.* MREA, Liverpool.

Roinn Oideachais (1971) Curaclam Na Bunscoile: Dublin S.O.

Ross, E.M., Peckham, C.S., West, P.B and Butler, N.R. (1980) Epilepsy in Childhood: findings from the National Child Development Study. *British Medical Journal* **1**: 207-210.

Ross, E.M., and Peckham, C.S. (1983) Seizure disorder in the National Child Development Study. In: *Research Progress in Epilepsy* (ed. F.C. Rose). Pitman Medical, Tunbridge Wells, pp.46-59.

Ross, E.M. and Tookey, P. (1988) Educational needs and epilepsy in childhood. In: *Epilepsy, Behaviour and Cognitive Function* (Eds. M.R. Trimble and E.H. Reynolds). John Wiley & Sons Ltd.

Royal College of General Practitioners (1992) *Epilepsy Information Folder.* RCGP Enterprises Ltd, London.

Rutter, M., Graham, P. and Yule, W. (1970) A neuropsychiatric study in childhood. *Clinics in Developmental Medicine*, Nos. **35-36**. Spastics International/Heinemann Medical, London.

Ryan, R., Kempner, K. and Emlen, A.C. (1980) The stigma of epilepsy as a self-concept. *Epilepsia* **21**: 433-444.

Sand, H. and Zalkind, S.S. (1972) Effects of an educational campaign to change employer attitudes towards hiring epileptics. *Epilepsia,* **13**, 87-96.

Sander, J.W.A.S. and Shorvon, S.D. (1987) Incidence and prevalence studies in epilepsy and their methodological problems: a review. *Journal of Neurology, Neurosurgery and Psychiatry* **50**, 829-39.

Sander, J.W.A.S., Hart, Y.M., Johnson, A.L. *et al.* (1990) National General Practice Study of Epilepsy: newly diagnosed epileptic seizures in a general population. *Lancet* **336**, 1267-71.

Santiago, M. and Niedermeyer, E. (1988) Racial factors and epileptic seizure disorders. *Journal of Epilepsy,* **1**, 31-33.

Schneider, J.W. and Conrad, P. (1980) In the closet with epilepsy, stigma potential and information control. *Social Problems* **28**: 32-44.

Schneider, J.W. and Conrad, P. (1986) Doctors, information and the control of epilepsy. In: *Epilepsy: Social Dimensions* (Eds. B. Hermann and S. Whitman) Oxford, Oxford University Press.

Schuler, M., Donati, F., Vella, S., Ramelli, G.P. and Vassella, F. (1997) School Performance and Social Integration of Epileptic Children. Paper Presented at European Congress of Epilepsy (R.D.S.) Dublin.

Scrambler, G. (1993) Coping with epilepsy. In: *A Textbook of Epilepsy.* (Eds. Laidlaw, J., Richens, A. and Chadwick, D.) Edinburgh, Churchill Livingstone.

Scrambler, G. (1994) Patient perceptions of epilepsy and doctors who manage epilepsy. *Seizure* **3**: 287-93.

Scrambler, G. and Hopkins, A. (1988) Accommodating epilepsy in families. In: *Living With Chronic Illness: The Experience of Patients and Their Families* (Eds. R. Anderson and M. Murray). London, Unwin Hyman.

Scrambler, G. and Hopkins, A. (1990) Generating a model of epileptic stigma: the role of qualitative analysis. *Social Science and Medicine*, **30:** 1187-94.

Shovran, S. (1987) Management of Epilepsy in Adults. *Medicine International* 2, 1874-9.

Sidenvall, R. (1900) Epidemiology In: *Paediatric Epilepsy* (Eds. M. Sillanpaa, S.I. Johannessen, G. Blennow and M. Dam) Wrightson Biomedical Publishing Ltd.

Seidenberg, M., Beck, N., Geisser, M. *et al.* (1986) Academic achievement of children with epilepsy. *Epilepsia* **27:** 753-759.

Sillanpaa, M. (1973) Medico-social prognosis of children with epilepsy: epidemiological study and analysis of 245 patients. *Acta Paediatrica Scandinavica*, Suppl. **237,** 2-104.

Sillanpaa, M. (1983) Social functioning and seizure status of young adults with onset of epilepsy in childhood. An epidemiological 20-year follow-up study. *Acta Neurologica Scandinavica*, **68** (supplement 96): 1-81.

Sillanpaa, M. (1990) Prognosis of children with epilepsy. In: *Paediatric Epilepsy*, (Eds. M. Sillanpaa, S.I. Johanessen, G. Blennow and M.Dam) Petersfield: Wrightson Biomedical.

Sillanpaa, M. (1992) Epilepsy in children: prevalence, disability and handicap. *Epilepsia* **33** (3) 444-449.

Sonnen, A.E.H. (1988) Acceptable risk in epilepsy. In: *Epilepsy and Society: Realities and Prospects.* (Eds. Canger, R. Loeber, J.N., Castellano F.). Amsterdam: Excerpta Medica.

Spelman B.J. and Griffin S. (1994) (Eds.) Conference Proceedings: Special Educational Needs. Issues for the White Paper. Dublin, Education Department, U.C.D. and Educational Studies, Ireland.

Spelman, B.J. and Kinsella, W. (2000) Recommendations for a National System of Special Education Provision with Specific Reference to Children with Autism. Submission to the Governmental Task Force on Autism, (Unpublished).

Stanley, P.J. and Tillotson, A. (1981) *Epilepsy in the Community.* Leeds, England, School of Social Studies, Leeds Polytechnic.

Statutory Instruments (1983) The Education Act, (Special Educational Needs) Regulations 1983. HMSO: London.

Stedman, J., Van Heyningen, R., and Lindsay, J. (1982) Educational underachievement and epilepsy. A study of children form normal schools, admitted to a special hospital for epilepsy, *Early Child Development and Care*, 9,1, 65-82.

Stores, G. (1973) Studies of attention and seizure disorders. *Developmental Medicine and Child Neurology* 15 376-382.

Stores, G. (1975) Behavioural effects of anti-epileptic drugs. *Developmental Medicine and Child Neurology* 17: 647-658.

Stores, G. and Hart, J. (1976) Reading skills of children with generalised or focal epilepsy attending ordinary school. *Developmental Medicine and Child Neurology* 18: 705-716.

Stores, G., Hart, J.A. and Piran, N. (1978) Inattentiveness in school children with epilepsy. *Epilepsia* **19:**169-175.

Stores, G. (1981) Problems of learning and behaviour in children with epilepsy. In: *Epilepsy and Psychiatry* (Eds. M.R. Trimble and E.R. Reynolds) London: Churchill Livingstone.

Su, B. (1986) *Taiwan's 400 Year History.* Washington, D.C.: Taiwanese Cultural Grassroots Association.

Sutherland, J.M. and Eadie, M.J. (1980) *The Epilepsies, Modern Diagnosis and Treatment.* London: Churchill Livingstone.

Tattenborn, B. and Kramer, G. (1992) Total patient care in epilepsy. *Epilepsia* **33**: (Suppl.) :28-32.

The Commission for the Control of Epilepsy and its Consequences (1977) *Plan for Nationwide Action on Epilepsy,* Vols. **I** and **II**, part 2. Washington, DC, U.S. Government Printing Office.

Temkin, O. (1971) *The Falling Sickness: A History of Epilepsy from the Greeks to the Beginnings of Modern Neurology.* John Hopkins University Press Ltd., London.

Temkin, O. (1994) *The Falling Sickness: A History of Epilepsy From the Greeks to the Beginnings of Modern Neurology.* John Hopkins' University Press Ltd.

Thompson, P.J. (1987) Education in Young Children and Young People with Epilepsy. In: *Epilepsy and Education,* (Eds. Oxley J., Stores G.), London, Medical Tribune Group.

Thompson, P., Huppert, F.A. and Trimble, M. (1981) Phenytoin and cognitive function: Effects on normal volunteers and implications for epilepsy. *British Journal of Clinical Psychology,* **20**, 3, 155-62.

Thompson, P.J. and Oxley, J. (1989) Social difficulties and severe epilepsy: survey results and recommendations. In: *Chronic Epilepsy, Its Prognosis and Management* (Ed. M.R. Trimble). Chichester, John Wiley and Sons.

Thompson, P. and Oxley, J. (1993) Social aspects of epilepsy. In: *A Textbook of Epilepsy* (Eds. Laidlaw, J., Richens, A., Chadwick, D.W.) Edinburgh: Churchill Livingstone.

Thompson, P.J., and Trimble, M.R. (1983) Anticonvulsant drugs, cognitive function and behaviour. *Epilepsia,* (Suppl.1): 555-563.

Thompson, P.J. and Upton, D. (1992) The impact of chronic epilepsy on the family. *Seizure,* **1**:43-48.

Trimble, E.H. and Reynolds, M.R. (1981) *Epilepsy and Psychiatry.* Churchill Livingstone, Edinburgh.

Trimble, M.R. and Thompson, P.J. (1984) Sodium valproate and cognitive function. *Epilepsia,* **25**, (Suppl. 1), S60-S64.

Trimble, M.R. (1988) Anticonvulsant drugs: mood and cognitive function. In: *Epilepsy, Behaviour and Cognitive Function.* (eds. M.R. Trimble, and E.R. Reynolds) John Wiley and Sons, Chichester, New York.

Tringo, J.L. (1970) The hierarchy of preference toward disability groups. *Journal of Special Education* **4**, 3, 295-306.

Tsuboi, T. (1984) Epidemiology of febrile and afebrile convulsions in children in Japan. *Neurology,* **34**, 175-181.

Tylor Fox, J. (1928) A census of epileptic people in Surrey. *Lancet,* **2**, 545-547.

United Nations (1999) United Nations' Convention on Children's Rights

Uutela, A. and Sillanpaa, M. (1985) Epilepsy and society. IV.Awareness and attitudes towards epilepsy in 1983 in comparison to 1977 in Finland. *Kansanterreystiet Julk M* **90**:1-72. (In Finnish with English summary). No.**132**.

Verity, C.M. (1995) Febrile convulsions. In: *Epilepsy.* (Eds. Hopkins A., Shorvon, S. and Cascino, G.) London, Chapman and Hall.

Vinning, E. P. G. (1987) Cognitive dysfunction associated with antiepileptic drug therapy. *Epilepsia*, **28**, Supplement 2, S18-S22.

Waizkin, H. and Stoeckle, J.D. (1976) Information control and the micropolitics of health care: summary of an ongoing research project. *Social Science and Medicine* **10**:263-270.

Wallace, S. (1994) Practical problems of epilepsy management in children. *Seizure*, **3**: 177-182.

Ward, F. and Bower, B.D. (1978) A study of certain social aspects of epilepsy in childhood. *Developmental Medicine and Child Neurology* Suppl. **39** Vol. **20**, No. 1.

West, C. (1983) Ask me no questions....A study of queries and replies in physician patient dialogues. In: *The Social Organisation of Doctor Patient Communication* (Eds. S. Fisher and A. Todd). Washington, DC, Center for Applied Linguistics.

Wilde, M. and Haslam, C. (1996) Living with epilepsy: a qualitative study investigating the experiences of young people attending outpatient clinics in Leicester. *Seizure* **5**: 63-72.

Wolf, P. (1998) Epilepsy in literature: doctors and treatment. *International Epilepsy News.*

Zielinski, J.J. (1974) Epileptics not in treatment. *Epilepsia*, **15**, 203-210.

Zeigler, R. (1981) Impairments of control and competence in epileptic children and their families. *Epilepsia* **22**: 339-346.